VETERINARY LEADERSHIP

MICHELE DRAKE, DVM

Founder, The Drake Center for
Veterinary Care (1992–Present)
Chief Veterinary Officer,
GeniusVets (2016–Present)
US

VETERINARY LEADERSHIP

A PRACTICAL GUIDE FOR PRACTICE OWNERS AND MANAGERS

WILEY

Published by John Wiley & Sons, Inc., Hoboken, New Jersey.
Published simultaneously in Canada.

For general information on our other products and services or for technical support, please contact our Customer Care Department within the United States at (800) 762-2974, outside the United States at (317) 572-3993 or fax (317) 572-4002.

Wiley also publishes its books in a variety of electronic formats. Some content that appears in print may not be available in electronic formats. For more information about Wiley products, visit our web site at www.wiley.com.

Library of Congress Cataloging-in-Publication Data applied for
Paperback ISBN: 9781394292424

Cover Design: Wiley
Cover Image: © Michele Drake

Set in 12/16pt GoudyStd by Straive, Pondicherry, India

SKY10090017_110624

Contents

Foreword

IN THE EXPANSIVE COLLECTION of literature on leadership, there are countless perspectives, ideas, and approaches. Yet, amidst the diverse wealth of resources available, there remains a timeless truth. *Regardless of the profession, leadership is not a mere title, position of authority, or a set of skills. It is a profound personal journey of growth, service, and influence, a path that can inspire and motivate us to reach new heights in our professional lives.*

In the time that I've spent immersed in the pages of this book on leadership in veterinary practices, I have been continuously reminded of the profound impact that effective leadership has on our teams and organizations as a whole. At its best, leadership is a force that not only shapes our teams and inspires change but also empowers us to enhance animal care and strengthen our relationships with clients. At a time when recruitment and retention of staff are at their most challenging, applying the principles Dr. Drake discusses can truly transform your practice – from growth potential to employee satisfaction and every business aspect in between.

The result of investing time and energy into effective leadership skills is far too valuable for veterinary leaders to ignore: Renewed potential for ourselves and our teams to lead professionally rewarding and financially successful careers as veterinary professionals.

In her writing, Dr. Drake highlights a particular foundational aspect of effective leadership: the importance of accountability. Just as we hold ourselves accountable for our clinical decisions and outcomes, we must also take ownership of our roles as leaders within our practices. First and foremost, we must hold ourselves accountable. When we demonstrate personal accountability and are answerable for our actions and results, the same desire to promote accountability will permeate through the entire organization and become ingrained in our whole team. When we place accountability at the forefront of our approach to leadership, we can better recognize responsibilities, set clear expectations, and create a sense of belonging within our teams.

Alongside accountability, Dr. Drake emphasizes the significance of mindset and attitude in shaping our approach to leadership. Our mindset – beliefs, attitudes, and perceptions that we hold – influences how we interpret and respond to challenges, setbacks, and opportunities, all of which are constant in a veterinary hospital. By developing a growth mindset that embraces learning, resilience, and continuous improvement, we grow our effectiveness as leaders while navigating the complexities of veterinary practice with greater confidence and adaptability, fostering a sense of hope and optimism.

I often hear people say, "I don't have time," or "I am too busy." These are default responses when we are faced with an overwhelming task or a challenging situation. However, as Dr. Drake points out, simply using this excuse and dismissing our responsibility is not acceptable. It's a mindset that will limit our team's potential and hinder our ability to grow and succeed. By falling back on these negative justifications, we relinquish control over our actions and allow circumstances to dictate our course. We effectively rein ourselves into a passive role in our own lives, and we will continue to live with mediocrity at best and often simply fail. While I understand that these may be your initial thoughts, I urge you to give this book a chance. It has the potential to transform your leadership skills and your career.

Instead of relying on avoidance of our shortcomings or problems, we must shift our mindset, recognize challenges as opportunities, and frame our vision through optimism and empowerment. Rather than using "I don't have time" as a cop-out, we can reframe our mindset and approach challenges with a proactive attitude. The mindset and narrative we adopt in our practices every day can catapult us to be successful leaders with a fulfilling career and a sense of purpose in our profession.

Dr. Drake's experience and insight show a critical paradox within the veterinary profession; while we meticulously hone our skills in critical thinking, problem-solving, and planning when it comes to medicine and surgery, we often overlook the application of these same concepts to leadership within our practices. As a result, we find ourselves navigating leadership challenges without the same clarity and precision that we bring to our clinical work, ultimately leading to frustration and inefficiency.

To address this, Dr. Drake demonstrates that veterinarians must apply the same rigor and discipline to leadership as we do to medicine and surgery. By integrating critical thinking, problem-solving, planning, accountability, and a growth mindset into our leadership practices, we can elevate the quality of care we provide to our patients, enhance the well-being of our teams, and foster a culture of excellence within our practices.

In these pages, you will discover not only practical strategies and principles for leading with excellence but also the heart and soul of leadership – the qualities of character, vision, and empathy that truly set exceptional leaders apart. Throughout the chapters, you will encounter stories of accomplishment and hardship, lessons learned from successes and failures, and the wisdom gleaned from those experiences.

As you embark on this journey of learning the meaning and impact of true and effective leadership, I encourage you to approach these insights with an open mind and a receptive heart. Allow them to challenge your assumptions, ignite your passion, and inspire you to become the leader you were meant to be. I can say without doubt that Dr. Drake's hope for this book is to serve as an example of guidance and inspiration on your own leadership journey, empowering you to make a meaningful difference within your team and start your path toward a professionally rewarding and financially successful career in veterinary medicine.

Rena Carlson, DVM
AVMA President 2023–2024

About the Author

Michele Drake, DVM, is the founder of The Drake Center for Veterinary Care, a 12-doctor small animal practice in Encinitas, CA. The Drake Center is renowned for the quality of care and service provided there and has been voted the best veterinary practice in San Diego eight times by *Ranch and Coast* magazine. Dr. Drake is a contributor to *Veterinary Economics*, *AAHA Trends*, and *DVM360*. She is a regular speaker at industry conferences, where she provides practice owners with guidance on how to build practices with strong teams, healthy cultures, and excellent business performance. She is also the co-founder and chief veterinary officer of GeniusVets, the leading veterinary marketing platform. Dr. Drake has two boys in college and lives in San Diego, CA, with her husband David, labrador Bentley, Jack Russel terrier Wilbur, and a little old cat named Ruby. When she's not working with her practice team, Dr. Drake enjoys wilderness travel and is also an avid mountain biker and a decent skier.

Acknowledgments

WHILE I USE THE first person often in the book, everything I have achieved in life comes from the love and support of many special people in my personal and professional life. Healthy relationships are the root of my personal happiness and my ability to achieve and be satisfied with life. A special thank you goes to many people along the way who are my family, my good friends, my business partners, and my colleagues.

This started with my mom and dad, who always supported me and formed my early understanding of healthy relationships and boundaries. My mom taught me to think independently and always try new things. My dad provided me with a great role model as an entrepreneur and was my trusted advisor while I was looking for a practice to buy in the first few years. My dad passed away in 2009, but I believe he is an angel who continues to watch over me.

To my two sons, Christopher and Matthew, who tolerated so many phone calls and stop-offs at the practice over the years: You have been my teachers in humility and love.

To my manager Chris, who started in our first hospital as a receptionist while she attended college and slowly became a major contributor to the growth and stability of The Drake Center: Your role modeling and understanding of our culture and mission helped to build our fabulous and talented support staff team.

To Dr. Kathy Boehme, my first associate and then partner of 25+ years: I thank you for your friendship and your vast contribution to the humanity of our practice. I looked to Kathy for her earthly wisdom so many times and was never disappointed. Her gifts have enriched my life.

To Kim Prunty, RVT, who worked with me in LA before agreeing to join me in Encinitas three months after I purchased my first practice: From the inception, you were my right hand in surgery and patient care. Kim continues to run our surgery team, and our doctors joke that we might have to close the hospital when Kim retires.

To Lorraine Holweg, Loree Cook, Peggy Gralish, and Arlene Penacho: You are the people I turn to in times of need for support and answers. Thank you all for your commitment to our mission and guidance on the leadership team over the years.

All of the doctors of The Drake Center bring their talents to fuse together to form the most capable and supportive team in veterinary medicine. Dr. Keala Shotwell, Dr. Jen Hamlet, Dr. Sarah Dilworth, Dr. Heather Kovacevich, Dr. Taylor Borsack, Dr. Katie Tiglio, Dr. Madison VanWorth, Dr. Kristie Leslie, and Dr. Janice Lee. Your dedication to your patients, clients, and each other is inspiring.

I am in a transition process now where I will leave the leadership team in the capable hands of Dr. Borsack, Dr. Dilworth, and Chris, as I move on to my next phase. I have no doubts that they will be able to surpass everything we started together.

I would also like to acknowledge the team of GeniusVets in providing the support and framework to accomplish this book. Both of my partners, David Hall and Harley Orion, encouraged my writing of this book as another way to serve our profession.

Harley, in particular, was my coach and writing muse. We spent many hours together on this project and his patience and skill in moving this forward were major impetus in completing this book. Special thanks to Emily Peck and Erin Herbert for their exceptional proofreading and editing expertise, and to Brandi Dupre for orchestrating the final details. This book was a collaboration of the GeniusVets team and they deserve much credit in this achievement.

About the Companion Website

The book is accompanied by a website:

https://vetpracticeleader.com/

1

Yes, There Is a Problem

Yes, there is a problem today in veterinary medicine.

No, it is not hopeless.

It's not the situation, but how we decide to view and think about it, that makes all the difference.

After one of my recent talks, a veterinarian (DVM) came up and told me she had just been to a seminar where they were discussing all of the stressors in veterinary medicine, how hard our field is, and how detrimental it is to mental health. She said she felt as if they were telling her "she should be feeling very bad and sad" about being a DVM and practice owner. She said she walked out of the talk and shook it off, saying to herself, "I have an amazing profession, an awesome practice, and a wonderful life" – and she was pretty annoyed that the message of the

Veterinary Leadership: A Practical Guide for Practice Owners and Managers, First Edition. Michele Drake.

seminar was so very negative. I love that she pushed back on this idea of victimhood and burnout. I agree with her. But it's unfortunate that she, and many other DVMs, are regularly having this messaging pushed on them at some of our biggest conferences. It's up to those of us with strong management skills to help out and mentor those who want to find this same place of love for our profession, for ourselves, and most definitely for our teams. We can do this.

We are navigating some difficult challenges and worrying trends in veterinary medicine today.

Of course, there's a significant shortage of veterinarians and trained technicians, with many DVMs retiring, and too few joining the profession to take their place.

Mental health and wellness concerns are being raised constantly. Even if you were not feeling particularly stressed before, the information you're seeing in most places is telling you that you *are* stressed, and that you are a victim of the current circumstances.

All of this is leading to an epidemic of "powerlessness" among many in our profession as Kogan and Rishniw[1] have found, which is creating many negative downstream effects – not the least of which is the corporate takeover of our industry – which does not appear to be to our benefit. But if you're in this profession, you don't need me to tell you this. You're already living it – or at least reading about it.

It's my personal mission to help change this current narrative and bring us back to seeing veterinary medicine as the amazingly fulfilling and wonderful career that it should be.

I believe veterinary medicine is more of a "calling" than a career. We are so lucky to have this opportunity to combine science, nature, and the beauty of the human–animal bond all into one career. I feel there has been far too much time dedicated to telling us what's wrong with our profession, and that we should all feel like victims. I would like to help change this narrative by sharing another way of looking at things – a way to elevate the circumstances of our workplaces and help more people have a fulfilling career in veterinary medicine. I believe our field is full of smart, caring humans who together can continue to make veterinary medicine one of the best ways to spend your professional life. I hope I can contribute to making a career in veterinary medicine a great one.

In this chapter, I'm going to address some of the key factors that I believe are actually leading to the difficulties in our profession today, and what I think underlies these issues. Then, in the remaining chapters, I will take you through what I've done to take on these challenges and build a successful practice – and I'll show you how you can do something similar in your own practice.

The Talent Shortage Meets the Pandemic Puppies

We've been shorthanded in Registered Veterinary Technicians (RVTs) and DVMs in some areas for a long time. But things got exponentially worse during COVID as a perfect storm converged:

- We all saw a tremendous increase in the need for our services during COVID. Different sources gave different reasons for this. I believe it was mostly that people were home 24/7 with their pets, and thus were more focused on the well-being of their pets and more likely to notice potential issues. This is a good thing – but it created an unexpected surge in demand.
- Dog breeders accelerated the pace of breeding, and many people looked to breeders and shelters to adopt dogs and cats to fill all of their free time.
- Older DVMs accelerated their retirement due to the challenges of delivering services during the pandemic.
- Managing the crush of the pet owner's needs and reduced staff availability was stressful.
- Enhanced unemployment made it difficult to retain entry-level staff, who could earn almost as much by *not* working.

In short, COVID drove a decrease in people available to work and a simultaneous increase in demand for our services.

Corporate Influences

The shift toward corporatization is also reshaping the landscape of veterinary care, as corporate groups often prioritize private equity returns and profits over quality of care. The animal care and pet industry has boomed over the last decade, with the industry now valued at nearly $150 billion,[2] and private equity firms and corporate investors have taken note. Research estimates that corporate veterinary practices account for approximately 10% of general companion animal practices and 40–50% of referral practices in the United States veterinary services market.[3] This problem has increased greatly as practice valuations have escalated, and very few associates (who usually carry significant student debt) are able to put together the capital needed to buy their practice from the original owner. In addition, most associates I've met are not interested in the lifestyle required of an owner. When you add in the fact that many practice owners are struggling with the current conditions – and all the propaganda saying practice ownership is stressful and ruins your mental health – you can't really blame an associate for not wanting to go down that path.

M&A Has Changed the Industry

Also, remember that corporations in our industry have gained more access to us by way of mergers and acquisitions. For example, many of our "industry media" and conferences, which were founded by DVMs or others not primarily motivated by profit, are now owned or controlled by commercial interests. So it can be difficult to ascertain who is actually speaking to us and what their motives may be. It can be hard to determine who their messaging and content really benefits.

Many of these corporate interests are regularly pitching us new products, services, or technologies that we now "must have." Being a leader means knowing what to say "no" to – even if just a "no for now." As a small business, you should choose your projects carefully, knowing what you and your team can manage well. And, remember, take "baby steps." You cannot do everything at once.

Data-driven corporations and technology platforms are aggressively pushing to marginalize the role of DVMs in the veterinary care process. They are skilled at leveraging financial capital with targeted marketing, public relations, and regulatory lobbying, all aimed at sidelining the veterinarian and making technology the center of pet healthcare. Legislation and lobbying efforts have been aimed at eroding the veterinarian–client–patient relationship (VCPR). Much of this legislation appears to be guided by corporate interests in order to monetize veterinary medicine by reducing the veterinarian's input into patient care.

Pet owners increasingly get pet care information online,[4] but the online environment is dominated by corporate players who are focused not on delivering quality information and steering pet owners to their local DVM, but rather on selling their raw food diets, Cannabidiol supplements, or telemedicine consultations to generate profits.

Care and Service Are Suffering

Poorly managed hospitals with weak leadership lead to unhealthy working environments for staff. Shorthanded teams mean longer wait times for clients. Overworked staff means more mistakes and risks to the well-being of our pets. Unhealthy practice environments lead to unhappy, stressed, unsupported staff. All this is legitimately frustrating for pet owners. Unfortunately, they often take out their frustrations on the very people who are trying to help them – DVMs and their staff. Whether through verbal abuse, one-star reviews, or social media rants sent around the world in an instant, these behaviors harm the hard-working and well-meaning people in veterinary medicine.

We need to do better. And we can.

Burnout and Wellness Challenges Have Escalated

If you were, or are, working in a poorly managed practice, all of the above issues have contributed to burnout. Burnout has become a common topic in every discussion in every veterinary forum.

But that's actually the problem: Too many people in veterinary medicine have accepted the idea that "this is how it is" and have stopped seeing this as irrational and wrong. Many have started to believe that burnout is a function of our industry.

It is not.

We need to change our perspective. We have an amazing profession where we serve our community by caring for animals. This should be a fulfilling and wonderful career – and it can be. The problem is not with the practice of veterinary medicine itself, but rather with the business around it – the administration and management of veterinary hospitals, the economic and human resources challenges connected with this, and the prevailing negative narrative surrounding veterinary work and well-being.[5] It doesn't have to be this way.

You Can Do Something About It – If You Decide To

Despite this grim picture, it's crucial to recognize that these challenges, while significant, are not entirely beyond our control as practice owners.

The trends in the profession, the influence of corporate money, and the demographic shifts in the United States may be out of your control – but what happens inside your four walls as a practice owner has *always* been up to you.

Along with these challenging trends, there's an even worse development that I've been following for years with some dismay. It's the worst of these problems because it prevents the others from being solved. That problem is the *victim mentality*.

As Eckhart Tolle said, "When you complain, you make yourself into a victim . . . change the situation, leave the situation, or accept it. All else is madness."[6]

Over my 30-year career in veterinary medicine, and through speaking around the country, I've had the opportunity to meet thousands of veterinary practice owners and to observe thousands more in my interaction with online groups and forums. I've witnessed an ever-increasing number of people focusing on the negatives in our profession. From practice owners complaining about their poorly behaved staff, to staff complaining about their mean clients, there seems to be a huge emphasis today on what's wrong with everyone else.

But as any decent therapist will tell you, seeing yourself as the victim of other people's bad behavior is self-destructive, and it impedes your power to impact the situation.

There will always be difficult staff. There will always be clients who give you a one-star review and bad-mouth you on social media – even when the negative outcome with their pet was completely their own fault. It's not the situation; it's how we see it and what we do about it that determines our own happiness and fulfillment.

We do have to deal with these challenges. But we don't have to be the victims of them.

Take Back Your Power

In this book, my goal is to help you take back your power as a practice owner. I know you can do this because not every practice is struggling. In fact, many are thriving. These successful practices don't struggle with recruitment. They are profitable, well-run businesses. Most importantly, they foster strong cultures with a clear sense of mission. They demonstrate that with the right approach, veterinary practices can not only survive, but flourish – even in these challenging times.

I'll be looking into many of these strategies and approaches throughout this book and, in particular, I'll discuss what I've found successful in my own practice and what I have learned from other great practice owners.

The key lies in focusing on the areas we can control and learning from those who've navigated these challenges successfully. With that approach, we can start to turn the tide for our practices and, over time, for the profession as a whole.

The Common Denominator

While there are a wide range of challenges facing our profession, after 30 years in practice leadership, I've come to realize that there's a common denominator underlying all these issues. Specifically, this is a factor that prevents practices from effectively dealing with the challenges they encounter, and it's simply this: *Most veterinary practices are not healthy organizations.*

Unhealthy organizations respond to challenges by caving in, blaming, or seeing themselves as victims.

Healthy organizations respond to these same challenges by rising to the occasion, supporting one another, and recognizing their capacity to succeed in any circumstance.

If we want to turn this profession around, we need to build healthy organizations.

Over the years, I've learned that a healthy organization is not just a lofty ideal; it's a practical and achievable goal. Healthy organizations are more resilient to external shocks, whether economic downturns or sudden technological changes (or even pandemics!). They are better equipped to adapt, evolve, and thrive, even in the most challenging times.[7] In addition, in a healthy practice, the owner feels he or she has a team to work with, and this greatly alleviates the day-to-day stresses that accompany practice life. Having an engaged team is also extremely important for the mental health of everyone in the practice.

Why do healthy organizations win, especially during times of change?

Healthy Organizations Have Stable Teams

One of the standout features of healthy organizations is their lower staff turnover and superior teamwork. A supportive and cohesive environment fosters loyalty and dedication, making these practices places where people genuinely want to work. This naturally eases the recruitment process, attracting quality professionals who are committed to their roles.

Healthy Organizations Deliver Better Care

Healthy organizations invariably deliver better medical care. With a team that is engaged, motivated, and stable, the quality of care provided to patients significantly improves. This not only benefits the pets we care for, but also enhances our reputation among pet owners.

Healthy Organizations Have Better Clients

Healthy organizations inherently attract better clients. They are less upset by the occasional problem client, and they have a client base that values and respects their services. This creates a more positive and fulfilling work environment for everyone involved. Of course, we get the occasional rude or difficult client at The Drake Center. But this type of client quickly realizes that our whole team supports one another, and they cannot play the staff off against each other, or do other dysfunctional things. So they can see they won't get anywhere with us by being mean or rude, and they will either start to treat the staff with respect or go be a difficult client for one of our competitors. Either way, it's fine by us.

Healthy Organizations Are More Financially Sound

Financial solvency is another hallmark of a healthy veterinary practice. Such organizations are not just surviving; they are financially sound, and they have the resources to be proactive in their recruitment and growth strategies. This financial stability opens doors to new opportunities and allows for strategic planning and development. The practice owner is not worrying about day-to-day cash flow, but is looking out into the future and planning for expansion. In addition, the team is well-paid, which means they are more likely to stick around.

You Can Do This

I wrote this book because I firmly believe that you, too, can build a healthy organization. I aim to guide you through this process, sharing the ten key strategies that have worked for me and many others.

Building Your Veterinary Practice Operating System (VPOS)

When I look at the difference between strong, healthy practices and struggling ones, one thing the strong practices have in common is that they have an *operating system* for their business. They don't manage by the "seat of their pants," solving any given problem a different way every day depending on their mood, or which way the wind is blowing. I call the approach I take in my practice the Veterinary Practice Operating System (VPOS), in a nod to the excellent book *Traction: Get A Grip on Your Business*,[8] which talks about a more general idea of an operating system that applies to any type of business.

Here's how I would define this:

> *A VPOS is a disciplined and structured way of running a veterinary practice. It keeps the practice 100% focused on the mission. It elevates patient care while building a strong culture and creating clarity for the owner, team, and clients. By doing the above, it helps deliver a consistent, excellent experience for everyone connected with the practice.*

If you happen to be reading this and are outside the veterinary profession, you could be forgiven for saying, "Wait, isn't that basically just part of what a business *is*? Doesn't every business have this?"

On the other hand, if you've been around the veterinary profession for a while, I think you'll agree that sadly *very* few veterinary practices really have this in place.

This is unfortunate because it's not actually that difficult to create a system like this, and it pays off spectacularly at every level, from your personal well-being to your financial future.

You too can build a VPOS.

Having seen the huge variety of types of practices – urban, suburban, rural, emergency, GP, luxury, economy, equine, small animal, exotic, and so on – I've realized that there really is no one VPOS that would work for everyone. But there is a system you can follow to create one that's as unique as your practice and will help you achieve your dreams in this profession.

That system is what I've outlined in this book.

Each of the following chapters is built around a specific value, mindset, or strategy that I've found to be successful. In each chapter, I'll explain the theory and thinking behind that lesson and how it can be applied in your practice. Then, at the end of the chapter,

I've provided specific exercises you can follow. The end product of each of these exercises is a component of your VPOS, so if you follow along, by the end of this book, you'll have created a more or less complete VPOS of your own.

I'm not here to say that my approach is the only correct one. In fact, I strongly encourage you to modify and adjust your VPOS however you see fit to make it perfect for your practice.

Ultimately, it's less about exactly what each detail of your system *is* and more about *having* a system that you follow. As your practice grows and changes, your VPOS will need to change and evolve as well.

My wish for you is that you become the best practice owner you can be and that you pass these lessons on to your team. Together, we can truly improve our businesses, elevate the quality of care, and leave this profession in better shape than we found it.

We can do this.

References

1. Kogan LR, Rishniw M. Veterinarians and moral distress. Journal of the American Veterinary Medical Association 2023;261(5):1–7.
2. Industry Trends and Stats [Internet]. (2023). American Pet Products Association. Available from: https://www.americanpetproducts.org/research-insights/industry-trends-and-stats
3. Nolan, R. The Corporatization of Veterinary Medicine [Internet]. avma.org. American Veterinary Medical Association; 2018. Available from: https://www.avma.org/javma-news/2018-12-01/corporatization-veterinary-medicine
4. Solhjoo, N., Naghshineh, N., and Fahimnia, F. The Internet and pet health: Case study of online health information seeking behavior of pet owners. Journal of Information Systems and Services. 2017;6(1–2):1–6.
5. Wallace, J.E. Meaningful work and well-being: a study of the positive side of veterinary work. Veterinary Record. 2019;185(18):571.

6. Tolle, E. The Power of Now: A Guide to Spiritual Enlightenment. New World Library; 2004.
7. Kriger, M., Zhovtobryukh, Y., Kriger, M., and Zhovtobryukh, Y. Creating truly healthy organizations in the long term. Strategic Leadership for Turbulent Times 2016;115–33.
8. Wickman, G. Traction: Get a Grip on Your Business. BenBella Books, Inc.; 2012.

2

Speaking from Experience

Always look at the source and learn to trust yourself and your instincts when receiving information and making decisions on how to run your practice.

When I look back to my 27-year-old self and think about what motivated me and inspired me, I find a few things that stand out. I love animals, and I was driven to provide the kind of care I would want for my own pets. And I wanted to manage a team who felt the same way. It really was that simple. The guidance and inspiration came from many places, but the key for me is knowing that I do not know everything, so I've continued to seek out people and information that bring value to my own journey. Eckhart Tolle says that if you really listen, then you know when you hear the truth. So always listen carefully and decide what resonates for you.

Veterinary Leadership: A Practical Guide for Practice Owners and Managers, First Edition. Michele Drake.
© 2025 John Wiley & Sons, Inc. Published 2025 by John Wiley & Sons, Inc.

Before we dig into the specific lessons and start building your VPOS, I feel it's important to establish why this approach is credible and worth considering.

I'll use a metaphor that will be familiar to most readers: After coming upon a case or a surgery that was especially challenging, or if the outcome was unknown, most of us would begin to search for some help and or answers. You might open a textbook by a doctor we trust, search on VIN, call a specialist, or read a veterinary journal. You would never just "guess" a solution and "muddle through it" as best you could. That would be malpractice!

But owning and running a practice can often be more difficult than seeing patients or doing surgery. *So why do we "muddle through" our challenges or ignore our problems instead of going to a proven, credible source and asking for help?*

I believe it is because, quite often, veterinarians simply don't know where to begin to make changes in their practice. I have owned a successful practice for over 30 years. I'm proud of many things about our practice, but the aspect I'm most proud of is that our doctors never leave unless they move away. And we have been financially successful for every one of these 30 years. This is not accidental. It takes a lot of work and thought, and a disciplined process, to create this type of practice. In this book, I am going to share my insight, wisdom (something you can only share after the age of 50!), and a process for you to create your own remarkable practice. But before we truly begin, it's important to understand that I didn't invent all this myself. I realized early on that I needed to look outside the veterinary industry to find great advice on leadership and business. So, I studied whatever I could get my hands on, and I applied it as best I could.

Two essential books that have played a pivotal role in shaping our operational framework are *Traction* by Gino Wickman and *The Five Dysfunctions of a Team* by Patrick Lencioni.

Traction provides an operating system that streamlines our day-to-day activities,[1] while *The Five Dysfunctions of a Team* offers insights into building a cohesive team.[2] Together, they form a powerful combination that any business, small or large, can benefit from.

Your Inputs Affect Your Results – What Are You Mentally "Feeding" Yourself?

In veterinary practice, as in any aspect of life, the information we consume significantly influences our attitudes and behaviors. This, in turn, shapes our actions and outcomes. It's crucial to be mindful of the *sources* and the *nature* of the advice we receive. Eckhart Tolle[3] once said, "You recognize the truth when you hear it." Tolle has been one of the many important influences in my life.

Choosing our sources of information wisely can be a game-changer. We succeed when we tune in to voices that not only educate, but also inspire positive changes. Seek out content that challenges you to think differently, encourages you to innovate, and offers specific actions to create improvement. Whether it's through books, seminars, online resources, or personal mentors, the goal is to find inspiration that drives positive transformations. I tend to see the "glass half-full." It's very important as an entrepreneur to see the world in a positive light. I cannot imagine being successful while having a victim or negative mentality.

Be Thoughtful About Who You Listen To – The Importance of Relevant and Proven Experience

When it comes to learning, be selective. The sources you turn to for information should not only inspire positive change, but also be accurate, reliable, and backed up with results.

The veterinary industry is replete with speakers and consultants who have little or no direct experience in running a veterinary practice. While their academic insights or external perspectives can be interesting and helpful, the lack of hands-on experience makes their advice less applicable – and sometimes even counterproductive. Just because someone writes an article or gives a talk at a conference, that doesn't mean their information is credible or right for your practice.[4] If you're intuitive, then you'll know what information is right for your practice and your team. In clinical practice, you wouldn't take advice on how to do a surgery from someone who has never done that surgery – we value practical and evidence-based experience highly.[5] The same principle should apply when seeking business advice. Seek guidance from those who have actually achieved success in running a veterinary practice.

Additionally, I'm interested in the experiences that have influenced their information. Whether it's a new surgical technique, business management strategy, or client communication approach, the key is to seek evidence-based information from people who have delivered results with that solution.

Every practice has a unique set of factors, including location, size, and distinct geographic qualities. All of these and more make our practices unique. Only we (the practice owners and team) can decide what is best for our practices.

Why I Think My Ideas Are Important Enough to Put Into a Book

With all of the above in mind, I'd like to share a little about my background.

Like many of you, I'm something of an introvert, and I really don't like talking about myself; so I'm going to keep this brief. But since I just outlined why it's vital to know where your inputs come from, I think this is important enough to share.

I grew up in St. Louis, Missouri, in an entrepreneurial family. My grandfather dropped out of grade school during the Depression and became a very successful real estate developer in St. Louis. My dad was a home builder who owned his own business, Drake Homes.

As a young girl, I followed my dad around in his truck and watched him deal with his customers and subcontractors. He was a very kind and ethical businessman. His customers referred him to their friends, and that's how his business grew.

Starting at age eight, I began to read *The Wall Street Journal* with my father. We would discuss business and economics throughout my childhood and young adulthood. I did not have any financial help after graduating from veterinary school, but my dad would still offer advice as I got started as a business owner. Those articles and columns have been important in forming my view of business and the world. I continue to begin each day with the ritual of a good cup of coffee and *The Wall Street Journal*. I read it daily and find it to be one of the only remaining reliable sources of good journalism and great information on economic trends and consumer habits.

All of this gave me a basic understanding that the decisions and actions of a business leader will determine their outcomes in the end. There will always be external factors in a business, but effective leaders find ways to accomplish their mission even when faced with challenges. In fact, I believe that challenging times are the most effective time to review all aspects of our business and position ourselves for greater success moving forward.

I graduated from the University of Missouri College of Veterinary Medicine in 1989. Because I grew up and went to school in the Midwest, I wanted to experience another part of the country when I graduated. I got a job and moved to Los Angeles to enjoy some sunny weather and play beach volleyball in my free time. I worked as an associate for three years. I learned a lot during that time, and I also discovered my passion and drive for providing the very best care and service. I felt I would never be able to completely fulfill this mission while working for someone else. So, at age 27, I bought my first practice in the little beach town of Encinitas, California.

Westlake Veterinary Hospital was a one-doctor and three-employee practice of 1,200 square feet. Within one year, I bought a second practice in a neighboring beach community, and finally, six years later, I purchased a third practice in Encinitas. This third practice purchase included a free-standing building. I bought the building and the practice and merged my little practices into this one to become The Drake Center for Veterinary Care.

Early on, my team and I created a mission statement. The culture developed naturally from the beginning. Within the first three months of owning the practice, I fired our only RVT because she wasn't nice to the other employees. I explained to the employees that I felt it was important that we have nice people who work together as a team. This showed them I was serious about creating a healthy and positive workplace. I recruited a replacement RVT who had worked for me in Los Angeles, and she's still with the practice today after 30+ years!

Later, as we grew, we defined specific core values for the practice as well. These have been valuable tools for hiring, training, and managing the practice.

The Drake Center for Veterinary Care
Mission Statement

To provide the best medical and surgical care in a compassionate environment for my patients and unsurpassed service for my clients.

This mission became the cornerstone of my practice. Everything we did for the next 30 years was to support this mission. It turns out that this is also a very good business plan.

The Drake Center Core Values
- Steadfast care and service
- Pursuit of excellence
- Compassionate partnership

To build the practice, I worked six days a week and took calls seven days a week. I raised my two boys during this time as well. It was an intense and often challenging road. When I encountered challenges I didn't know how to solve, I studied, looked for mentorship, and leaned on my team to help find answers. One thing that I quickly realized was that there isn't a lot of great information about business management within our profession. So I often turned to classic leadership books that are familiar to many business leaders, but sadly pretty unknown in our profession – books like *Traction: Get a Grip On Your Business* by Gino Wickman, *The Five Dysfunctions of a Team* by Patrick Lencioni, and *The Effective Executive* by Peter Drucker. I also became a member of Veterinary Management Groups (VMG), where I was able to connect with other high-quality practice leaders who were similarly committed to delivering great medical care while also running a great business. The other practice owners in my VMG group became some of my best friends.

Over the last 30 years since my initial steps in the profession, we've grown The Drake Center from a single-doctor practice to a team of 12 veterinarians, supported by a dedicated staff of 55. With the help of my manager, excellent leadership team, and staff, the practice has expanded significantly even during the challenging times of COVID-19, achieving over 35% growth and opening a second annex location.

I don't want to spend a lot of time talking about my lifestyle because I've seen a lot of "gurus" and "influencers" who make far too big a deal about theirs. But I do think it's important to discuss because I know many practice owners struggle with their lifestyle – overworked, never taking a vacation, and sometimes feeling like "their practice owns them."

Because I've created a disciplined operating system and built a strong, aligned, and dedicated team, I have been able to work *on* my business rather than *in* my business for many years. I have not needed to be in clinical practice regularly for 10+ years (though I did step in from time to time during COVID). My practice thrives and stays true to our mission even when I'm not in the building. This has enabled me to spend uninterrupted time raising my two boys; to take life-changing trips to Alaska, Africa, and Europe; to lean into my wellness through competitive downhill mountain biking; and so much more. While it took hard work to get here, I have achieved a level of freedom and resources that is truly wonderful, and I want that for each one of you. And it's not just me – many doctors of veterinary medicine who are my close friends have achieved amazing lifestyles by applying similar strategies. Taking on the risk and challenge of business ownership should come with great rewards in time. Don't miss out on them.

While I use the first-person "I" and "we" interchangeably in this book, I did not accomplish much of anything alone. When I bought my first practice, I inherited a young receptionist, Christine Spencer, who developed into our hospital manager. I often refer to her as the "heart and soul of our practice" because she exemplifies our culture and is dedicated to our staff and clients. Her deep understanding and stalwart support of our mission have been keys to moving us forward in every endeavor. In addition, she provided me with a constant sounding board for my visions and plans. My first associate, Dr. Kathy Boehme, became my only partner after working with me for five years. I always joked that we took turns having our kids to make sure that one of us was full-time in the practice during the other's maternity leave. This set the tone for future associates having children and raising kids while working at The Drake Center. We have always stood for families first and supported each other in times of need. Dr. Boehme is also at the heart of our practice, pushing constantly to create the utmost in relationship building with our teams and our clients. There are so many others who have made massive contributions to building The Drake Center, and I am grateful to all of them.

Today, I'm also a nationally recognized speaker, sharing my experiences and insights with hundreds of other practice owners every year. I speak on creating healthy organizations, cultivating positive cultures, building strong teams, and attracting and retaining top talent. I've served on boards for leading veterinary pharmaceutical companies and have worked closely with our leading certifying organizations and trade associations. I have no interest in being in the spotlight, but I would like to share some of the wisdom and experience I've accumulated as I begin to shape the next chapter in my life. I'm not starting a consulting company and I don't want to be a "guru." I simply want to share what I've learned. I hope it resonates with many of you and helps you make your practice stronger.

This book isn't for me – it's for you. I firmly believe that success in veterinary practice is attainable for anyone with the discipline and commitment to put in the work. I am living proof that, with the right mindset and approach, remarkable achievements are within reach.

Many of the lessons in this book are probably different from what you've been hearing around the industry. But if you really look around, I think you'll agree that our industry isn't in the best shape – so maybe some different ideas are needed.

Let's Get Started

Ok, that's enough about me. Let's now turn our focus to the 10 lessons I've learned in building and leading my practice. These lessons have enabled me to make it a great success, providing an amazing lifestyle for myself and my family, a great workplace for my team, and the best source of care and support for pet owners and pets in my community.

References

1. Wickman, G. Traction: Get a Grip on Your Business. BenBella Books, Inc; 2012.
2. Lencioni, P. The Five Dysfunctions of a Team. San Francisco, CA: Pfeiffer; 2002.

3. Tolle, E. The Power of Now: A Guide to Spiritual Enlightenment. New World Library; 2004.
4. Wales, T. Practice makes perfect? Practicing veterinarians' information seeking behaviour and information use: implications for information provision (Doctoral dissertation, C).
5. Leachman, C. LibGuides: Veterinary Medicine: Resources for Practicing Veterinarians (EBVM) [Internet]. libguides.libraries.wsu.edu. Available from: https://libguides.libraries.wsu.edu/veterinary medicine/EBVM

3

Accountability

When something isn't working, point the finger at yourself, not others.
"The bad news is, it's up to you ... and the good news is, it's up to you."

When you become a practice owner, there are so many decisions you'll have to make. It will be exhausting at times. However, don't take the "easy way out" and just do what makes you popular or more liked.

Within the first few months of my first practice, I had to eliminate all the discounts that my predecessor had started. I didn't have a trust fund, and I owed a lot of money to the bank, so to a degree, this was an economic necessity. But in addition to that, I couldn't find any reason why I should give discounts, as my mission was always to provide the best care.

Veterinary Leadership: A Practical Guide for Practice Owners and Managers,
First Edition. Michele Drake.
© 2025 John Wiley & Sons, Inc. Published 2025 by John Wiley & Sons, Inc.

I cannot do that while also providing discounts. So, I stopped them all, and I received intense pushback from some clients. I was 27 and a new business owner, and I clearly remember a few very intimidating conversations with a group of Harley-Davidson bikers that my predecessor used to give discounts to. It still makes me sweat today thinking about it. But I was accountable to myself, my team, my patients, and also to the bank. When you have a sound reason for making decisions, remain accountable to them. This will make the rest of the decisions somewhat easier. When you follow your mission, it will be clear what the decision should be.

Everything Begins with Accountability

I feel very fortunate that I've had such a successful career in veterinary medicine, but I'm troubled by all the struggles I see my peers going through. Many of the things I've done to achieve my goals as a practice owner were simple – but not easy.

I'm certainly not perfect, and I'm sure there are practice leaders out there who are even better than me in some of these areas. But I do have one trait that I think helped me build all the rest, and that really created the trajectory of my career. That trait is *personal accountability*.

When I tell my team I am going to do something, I do it. When we decide upon our culture, we adhere to it. When we train for new skills, we follow up to make sure they are being used.

A great place to start with accountability is in your decision to have a strong mission statement and be accountable to this mission statement in everything you do. When I hire new staff members, I tell them about the history of the hospital. I want them to hear from me that our mission is to provide the best medicine and surgery in a compassionate environment and unsurpassed customer service for our clients. I tell our new employees that everything I've done, and that all of us do, goes to support this mission. I use our mission statement as a litmus test for every decision I make.

In the following chapters, I'm going to share key lessons and strategies that helped me, and I'll provide action plans to help you implement them in your own practice.

But before you can really start taking action toward your goals, you need to make a decision:

Going forward, who will be in charge of what happens in your practice?

As the practice owner (or manager or medical director), you must be willing to be responsible for everything that happens in your practice, good and bad. Of course, external challenges will come up – none of us will ever forget COVID-19 – but you always have the ability to choose how you respond to these challenges, and your choices and actions will ultimately determine your results.

I hope you will make the decision to be fully accountable for your practice so that you can get it moving in the right direction through these lessons.

What Is Accountability Really?

Accountability is not just a buzzword; it's the cornerstone of success, and today's leaders, especially in medical settings, are challenged more than ever to be accountable.[1]

I've noticed some people have a complicated idea of what accountability is. But the core concept is simple yet powerful: *When something isn't working, point the finger at yourself rather than others.* Take ownership of your business and have the courage to make the necessary changes without making excuses.

I often tell other practice owners that when it comes to fixing problems in your practice, "the *bad* news is, it's you ... and the *good* news is, it's you." At first, it might be uncomfortable to see yourself as the source of problems in your business, but in reality, it's tremendously empowering. It means that if there's anything about your practice you don't like or you think needs to be better, you can change it!

One place this comes up often is with practice culture and behavioral rules. I often find myself advising practice owners that if you have a good culture, but some people on your team aren't accountable for following your culture, it's your responsibility to address the issue – up to and including firing that person.[2] If you do not have a defined culture, then it's up to you to work with your team and shape your culture so people inside the building can all reach their potential. If you haven't yet gotten that in place, that's fine – but start now because it's very important! People can't really be held accountable for values they haven't been told about. I provide more guidance on creating a strong culture in subsequent chapters.

I've found that most practice owners are somewhere on a continuum from slightly conflict-averse to *very* conflict-averse, and this can really hurt your business. We all got into this business because we love science and animals. For most of us, this means we're often much more comfortable dealing with animals than with humans. So we tend to shy away from direct confrontation with humans, and this can cause us to allow problem behavior to go on for too long. Deep down, the business owner usually knows what really needs to be done.

It's a tough pill to swallow, but an important one. True progress will be hindered unless you reconnect with your mission and values, leverage them to make those difficult decisions, and refuse to make excuses. Accountability is about recognizing that either you already know the answer, or you can work with your team, or your mentors, or go research the answer yourself. Drop "I can't" and "I don't know how" from your vocabulary as a business owner, and you will greatly increase your success potential.

Embracing Accountability – Overcoming the Fear of Tough Decisions

I've found many practice owners are reluctant to really "take the reins," even when they know what needs to be done. Many of these decisions are "simple but not easy."

This is extremely common in personnel issues, for example. Many colleagues have approached me after my talks, acknowledging that they know they should part ways with an underperforming or disruptive employee – someone who affects the harmony of the team. Yet, they give a bunch of reasons why it's seemingly "impossible" to take that step. They'll say things like, "But I can't fire Jane; I know she's mean to the other staff, but she's my most experienced tech." This is a classic problem of accountability. As the owner, no one but you should be in control here, and you need to take on that responsibility and make the hard decisions needed for your practice to thrive. As a leader, your approach to decision-making sets a precedent for your organization and will determine its culture over time. Putting your organization's success and health above self-interest and excuse-making is imperative for ethical and sustainable leadership.[3]

In reality, what's harder? The challenge of making a tough call? Or letting this person continue to wreck the harmony of your practice? This is a simple decision, though not an easy one. Breaking free from dysfunction is the path to a healthier, more functional team. And we owe it to our team to provide them with the healthiest work environment possible.

I've seen a similar pattern with adjusting prices. With inflation and changing market conditions, we may have to raise prices at times to ensure fair compensation for the team and profitability for the business. Many DVMs tell me they're afraid of a client backlash, or they don't know how to explain the changes to their team so that they can discuss them with clients. But if you properly communicate why a change is necessary and how it aligns with the greater goals of the business and, ultimately, the well-being of patients, you can get everyone on board. We cannot control the economy – but we *can* control how we respond to it.

The two things that help keep your team on board with how you run the practice are:

1. Build a strong culture and let them know you will always champion this so they have the best workplace possible.
2. Communicate the state of your practice frequently.

Employees need to be made aware of *where you are now, where you're headed,* and *how you plan to get there.* In the absence of this type of communication, people make up their own stories that are rarely true and never benefit the team or your process.

Don't Plan to Fail

I often encounter a mindset where the practice owner has already decided a change is bound to fail:

"Clients will stop coming if I raise prices."

"If I ask that doctor to follow our new medical guidelines, they will get mad and quit."

"I know Mrs. Meanypants always yells at our staff, but if we don't give her what she wants, she'll write another bad review!"

This is called a "self-fulfilling prophecy." People like to be right. If you've convinced yourself a new idea won't work, chances are it won't. Accountability lies in acknowledging that, yes, it's a bold step and a bit uncomfortable, but it's a step toward progress and growth.

After my talks, people frequently approach me with a litany of reasons why my suggestions won't work in their specific situations.

They usually have a laundry list of reasons why. In response, I find myself asking, "What do you want me to do about that?" There's actually nothing I can do in that situation because *the decision has already been made* – the owner has "decided" not to make things better in their business and resigned themselves to their perceived limitations. It sometimes seems like they're looking for me to agree with them that nothing can be done about their situation. But that would not be honest. *There's always something the practice owner can do to turn things around.*

Accountability lies in challenging these self-imposed limitations and being bold in your decision-making. If you've fostered a collaborative environment within your team, where everyone is on board with sound decisions, the journey becomes less arduous. Teamwork, after all, is the linchpin of effective decision-making. So, as we work to increase accountability, let's do it without self-doubt and embrace the transformative power of bold, informed choices.

Take Baby Steps

A common stumbling block in our industry is the perception that thinking about practice management takes up too much time – time that could be spent in the exam room or performing surgeries. The truth is that it doesn't require a huge amount of time; it just demands focus and thoughtfulness. Prioritize the essential aspects of practice leadership and understand that change doesn't happen overnight.

Whether it's tackling marketing initiatives or addressing personnel issues, take it one step at a time. Schedule regular meetings, invest time in strategic planning, and witness the gradual transformation. You can't do everything at once, but consistent effort yields results.[4] It's the "baby steps" that eventually lead to significant progress.

Managing a veterinary practice is not just about the day-to-day clinical tasks. It's about thoughtful leadership, effective communication, and a willingness to evolve. By stepping back, reflecting on your purpose, engaging with your team, and taking measured steps, you'll find that the seemingly massive challenges become manageable, and positive change becomes easier.

Incorporating Accountability into Hiring and Training Processes

Accountability in the workplace begins with hiring people who fit into or add to our culture. The team is accountable for training well, and the new employee is accountable for taking appropriate steps to become proficient in their new role.

At The Drake Center, we prioritize hiring individuals who align with our organizational culture. During interviews, we assess not only the candidate's qualifications but also their values and compatibility with our team. Our hospital manager, skilled in fostering open conversations, plays a crucial role in gauging the cultural fit of potential team members. She is gifted in letting people talk about themselves with open-ended questions. This gives her great insight into who might fit our culture.

Once a candidate joins our team, it is up to the team to mentor, train, and make the new employee feel welcome. It starts with clear expectations regarding their training. We communicate the direction we intend to take with their development and outline specific tasks and milestones they are expected to achieve.

We provide new team members with a roadmap detailing the specific training videos they need to watch, the skills they need to acquire, and the individuals they will work with. This sets a tone of shared responsibility from the beginning of their tenure. While they may not be fully integrated into the team initially, we expect them to be accountable for their individual training tasks and proactive in completing their training.

We employ a system of continuous feedback and follow-up. We recently added the use of an app that includes the training process, the materials, and outlines for weekly tasks, ensuring clarity on what needs to be accomplished. Team members work with different individuals during their training to acquire diverse skills, preventing any one person from bearing the entire burden of training new employees. We actively seek feedback from the teams and doctors working with the new team members to assess their progress, skills, and overall helpfulness.

We encourage new team members to take personal inventory and reflect on their progress regularly. If expectations are not met, we initiate constructive conversations to understand the reasons and provide guidance for improvement. This approach emphasizes personal responsibility for their own development.

Accountability and Staff Retention

Accountability is pivotal in steering your team toward success. Staff turnover is a growing challenge for owners. According to the American Animal Hospital Association, annual turnover among veterinary staff is at 23%, and increasing steadily year over year.[5] Over the years, I've encountered staffing challenges that demanded a thorough examination of our own decisions and actions – and ultimately, accountability from leadership figures.

As one example, when faced with the need to part ways with an employee, the focus should be on evaluating ourselves, not on blaming the individual.

If an employee is not performing, either we *hired wrong* or we *trained wrong*. Those are the only two reasons. It's usually training. Everyone learns at a different pace. We will always work with individuals who fit our culture, persisting in training or moving them around to find a better position for their skill set. I have only ever fired one person ever for making mistakes. For any other team members that have been fired over the years, it was because they refused to fit into our culture and were disruptive to our mission.

Letting go of an employee is not a matter of fault-finding. Instead, it's an opportunity for reflection on three critical aspects: hiring the right person, placing them in the right role, and providing effective training. These considerations form the bedrock of a thriving team.

During a recent challenging hiring phase, we brought on board a genuinely nice individual who truly fit our culture. However, we soon realized that her skill set didn't precisely align with tasks demanding strong follow-through and attention to detail – qualities crucial in the role she had been put into. Instead of hastily letting her go, we decided to reassess her role.

Recognizing her strengths, we crafted a unique position within our surgery team. She became an invaluable part of tasks like chart documentation, post-dental charting, patient movement, surgical instrument preparation, and precalls for surgery clients. This tailored role allowed her to contribute value to the team without the burden of specific responsibilities that didn't match her skill set. It was a creative solution that preserved her place on the team, and it has been working very well. Similar conversations within the veterinary industry surrounding giving employees autonomy through allowing them to have input in aligning their roles with their interests and skill sets[5] have pointed toward increased job satisfaction and an increased likelihood of employee retention.

Not every situation unfolds as smoothly. There are times when, despite our best efforts, a team member doesn't align with the culture or exhibits behavior fundamentally incompatible with our values. In one instance, a seasoned technician voiced concerns about a colleague, who had been with us for almost three months, describing her as simply "a mean person." It wasn't just a matter of inadequate training; it was a question of character.

In such cases, quick action is needed. Trusting the feedback of my technician, who had observed the individual's behavior consistently even after multiple attempts to coach her, we made the difficult decision to part ways. In this case, it wasn't a failure of training; it was a realization that we had hired someone whose values did not align with our practice. Recognizing this, we took ownership of our mistake and terminated her employment after a few months.

The key takeaway from these experiences is the importance of constant evaluation and adaptability. Acknowledging mistakes, whether in hiring or training, is part of the learning curve. It's not just about finding the right people; it's about cultivating an environment where everyone can thrive. So, when faced with tough decisions, remember to look inward, talk to key members of your leadership team, and form a consensus based on supporting your mission and culture.

The Ripple Effect of Accountability

As a practice owner, defending and protecting your culture is a significant responsibility. When team members witness that their concerns are taken seriously and acted upon, it fosters trust and strengthens the team's bond.

In instances where a team member has to be let go due to cultural misalignment, for example, this underscores your commitment to maintaining a workplace where respect and professionalism are non-negotiable. I've had practice owners tell me they are "too nice" to fire employees. But this is just wrong: By not confronting problem employees or letting them go, you're not really being "nice" – you're actually disrespecting the rest of the team and degrading your culture.

How Accountability Benefits Cohesiveness

Building a cohesive and effective veterinary team is no small feat. None of us are doing this work for the "short hours and high pay." It's a tough job. And unfortunately many of the roles in a veterinary practice simply don't pay enough for people to do them while also being disrespected or mistreated.

I've always believed that fostering an environment of accountability plays a pivotal role in building a strong team. Leadership must always take responsibility, especially when things don't go as planned.

When a team witnesses its leadership owning up to mistakes, it sets a powerful example. Acknowledging vulnerabilities and addressing our own shortcomings creates a sense of unity. When leaders don't embrace accountability and shift responsibility for their errors, the consequences can be harmful to an entire team and affect employee perceptions of their leadership and workplace culture.[6] I make a conscious effort to handle any negative situation quickly, encouraging the team to confront issues head-on and then move forward. I firmly believe in dealing with challenges internally and avoiding unnecessary gossip or dwelling on setbacks. This also provides an example of setting boundaries, which we will discuss later in this book.

Accountability, Leadership, and Change

Your team looks up to you for guidance, and if changes are needed, it's the leader's responsibility to drive that transformation.

I've had the privilege of taking over three veterinary practices, each with its unique challenges. In these situations, I've been unapologetic about making tough decisions to ensure that the team aligns with the practice I want to create.

When I acquire or hire new team members, especially doctors, I make it crystal clear what our culture is all about. The response has been overwhelmingly positive, with the majority eager to be part of our unique and uplifting environment. While we're far from perfect, the palpable sense of camaraderie is evident to anyone who walks through the doors of The Drake Center.

Cultivating Accountability Across the Team

As a leader, your focus extends beyond your own accountability to nurturing this ethos throughout the entire team.

At the core of our strategy at The Drake Center is our leadership team. Within our leadership, we utilize something called the Traction System, which is a framework designed to align everyone within the organization with common goals. Documented in Gino Wickman's *Traction: Get A Grip On Your Business*, the Traction System is derived from the six major components of the Entrepreneurial Operating System (EOS):

1. Vision
2. People
3. Data
4. Issues
5. Process
6. Traction

At its core, the Traction System helps teams focus on business processes through two primary focuses: thorough documentation of key processes and adherence to these processes on an organizational level. This approach promotes ownership of key business functions and allows for greater accountability for team follow-through.[7]

In my practice, the Traction System is not exclusive to the leadership team; we ensure that every member of our staff has specific goals and responsibilities. Regular check-ins are a forum for discussing progress, identifying challenges, and collectively working toward our shared objectives.

Accountability isn't just about achieving strategic goals; it's about the everyday behaviors that contribute to a positive and efficient work environment. If someone on the team consistently shows up late, I don't shy away from addressing the issue directly. I approach the individual respectfully, seeking to understand the reasons behind their tardiness. By doing so, I emphasize the impact on the team and the importance of respecting everyone's time. In addition, this may be an opportunity to find out this person is having some tough times and may need some additional support.

In team meetings and leadership discussions, I emphasize that every action, including being punctual, plays a role in supporting our mission of providing the best medicine and surgery, and unsurpassed customer service. When someone shows up late, it contradicts our culture of respect, kindness, and trust. It's not about me being personally annoyed with them; it's about how their individual actions align with, or detract from, the shared values of the team and our ability to deliver on our mission.

Beyond the immediate workplace context, I make it clear to every team member that the habits and skills we instill are not just about the job at hand. These are life skills with enduring value. Punctuality, respect for others' time, and understanding the ripple effects of one's actions contribute not only to the success of our team but also to personal growth and success in any career. In other words, when you train a team member to be accountable, you are truly contributing to their long-term growth, both personally and professionally.

Instilling a culture of accountability involves weaving it into the fabric of everyday interactions, aligning individual efforts with collective goals, and fostering a sense of responsibility that transcends the workplace.[8] It's about creating a team that understands the broader impact of their actions and is committed to upholding the values that define your mission.

Personal Accountability in a Collaborative Setting

Success and challenges are shared experiences. While there may be instances when an individual's mistake is the obvious cause of an issue, it's usually best to focus on the bigger picture.

While it's easy to attribute failures to individual mistakes, the reality is usually more complex, and "human error" is not usually about that one human, but about a systemic way things are organized that creates an opportunity for things to go wrong.

For example, a specific tech knocked a pulse oximeter off a counter and broke it. It's easy to get frustrated with that team member. But if you take a step back, you might ask: *Was this piece of equipment placed in the best location? Was the counter wide enough? Does this treatment room have enough space for people and animals to move during busy times without bumping into each other or knocking things over?*

In other words, there's usually more to any situation than the most immediate circumstances. Recognizing this allows you to prevent future problems. Before the next piece of equipment gets knocked over, maybe someone should take a walk around the hospital and look for things that could be stored or positioned better.

This approach has a powerful effect on employee morale. When that employee just knocked over the pulse oximeter, if they've had a lot of mediocre bosses in the past, they probably expect to get yelled at. When instead, their boss asks what happened and points out that maybe that counter is too narrow or we should move these boxes to make the space safer or asks the employee if they have an idea of how we could avoid this in the future; it shows that their boss and managers truly have their back, and are not in a rush to assign blame.

In my hometown of San Diego, we had a severe two-day power outage, sometimes called "the Great Southwest Blackout of 2011."[9]

The way I remember it being reported on the news, some person in a power facility "pushed the wrong button" and caused a catastrophe. But this just begs the question – why is there a button you can push incorrectly that will knock out power to the entire Southwest? As it turns out, the story was a lot more complex – apparently, there were 23 distinct events that led to the blackout. There were multiple "single points of failure" that had existed for many years, and we just got lucky up until that one moment, when a seemingly simple action led to widespread consequences.

When something does go wrong, look for the systemic causes rather than simply blaming the person who might have just been in the "wrong place at the wrong time." No employee has ever been yelled at in The Drake Center – and no one ever will be.

When you approach problems this way, taking full responsibility as the owner for creating the conditions that lead to safety – or to mishaps – it creates a similar commitment in your team. They will start to spot potential problems before they happen and help prevent them.

If a decision or strategy isn't yielding the expected results, we acknowledge that we made the choice as a team. This enables us to collaboratively address the issue, whether it involves reevaluation, training, or adjustments in our approach.

The Impact of Accountability on Client Experience

Accountability extends far beyond internal operations; it profoundly influences the experience your clients have with your practice, as well as the quality of the medical care you provide.

One key aspect of accountability, as perceived by our clients at The Drake Center, is our unwavering commitment to follow through on every aspect of their pet's care. Whether it's an emergency situation or a routine visit, we prioritize thorough documentation and communication. If a critical care facility becomes necessary, we ensure that all information is seamlessly transferred, and we take the initiative to follow up with the client the next day. This proactive approach reassures our clients that we are not merely providing the service they are paying us for, but are truly dedicated to the entire journey of their pet's well-being.

Our commitment to accountability includes setting clear expectations for the quality of care we provide. When clients observe our team's behavior, from the initial consultation to ongoing follow-ups, they understand that we go beyond "quick fixes." We don't just apply a temporary solution; we commit to seeing a case through to its resolution. If a surgery doesn't go as planned or a treatment is not yielding the expected results, our approach is not to hope the issue fades away. We actively engage with the situation, following up with clients and taking necessary steps to address concerns.

For new team members, witnessing this level of accountability can be eye-opening. The realization that we actively follow up with clients, regardless of the situation, creates a standard for how care is expected to unfold. Whether it's ensuring a postsurgery call or addressing issues that arise, our team understands that accountability is not just a buzzword but a tangible part of our professional behavior.

Technology Does Not Replace Accountability

In an era dominated by technological tools and innovations, I want to emphasize the irreplaceable value of human-to-human interaction. While new technology tools, such as digital record systems, online appointment scheduling, and telemedicine, may enhance certain aspects of our workflow, it's crucial to discriminate between tools that genuinely contribute to efficiency and those that merely add complexity. The core of our accountability lies in the personal connections and collaborations within the team, which remain paramount for excellent patient care.

There is a lot of push for technology from every place you look (or listen). Please remember to follow your instincts. Investigate, review, and consult with others in your practice and outside of your practice.

Nurturing a Culture of Accountability Through Continuous Investment

Building a culture of accountability is not a one-time endeavor[8] – it requires continuous investment, commitment, and a proactive approach.

One place that we've worked to increase accountability is to better understand the drivers of turnover. Some turnover is inevitable in the veterinary field, especially with the influx of young professionals who are just "checking out" our field and are not sure if they will pursue it as a career. The sooner you accept this and take responsibility for making a plan to handle it, the better. Rather than viewing turnover as a hurdle, embrace it as an opportunity to differentiate your practice from others by creating ongoing training and skill development programs.

Embrace the reality that training is a constant. Your leadership team is integral to this mindset shift. Recognize that ongoing training is not just a necessity but a strategic investment in the growth and success of the practice.

The challenge lies in making training dynamic, efficient, and successful.

Utilizing a combination of mentorship, in-house videos, and external resources offers an interactive learning experience. Visual elements complement hands-on practice, ensuring that team members grasp concepts comprehensively. Providing diversity in training tools will serve not only to educate but also to energize the learning process. Current research supports this approach and suggests the implementation of varied training materials and reinforcement through discussion and testing.[10]

The Benefits of Embracing Accountability

Practice owners stand to gain huge advantages by embracing accountability within their practices. This transformative approach alleviates the burden on owners and propels the entire team toward continuous improvement. Here are several key benefits that practice owners can reap by applying this invaluable lesson:

Shared Responsibility

By instilling accountability throughout the practice, the onus is no longer solely on the owners. A culture of accountability involves the entire team, distributing responsibility and fostering a collective effort toward achieving practice goals.

Effective Planning

Accountability requires a clear understanding of where the practice is headed. Practice owners benefit from involving the entire team in strategic planning, tapping into diverse perspectives, and creating a unified vision that guides decision-making.

Enhanced Success

As accountability becomes ingrained in the practice culture, owners witness a surge in performance. The positive ripple effect extends beyond the practice walls to benefit pet owners and their beloved pets. Here's how.

Elevated Patient Care

A commitment to continuous improvement directly impacts patient care. As the practice evolves and refines its approaches, patients receive enhanced medical attention, ensuring that their well-being is prioritized at every stage.

Cutting-Edge Care

Embracing accountability propels practices to stay informed about the latest advancements in veterinary medicine. Owners and team members engage in ongoing education, ensuring that they remain at the forefront of industry developments and offer cutting-edge services.

Transparent Communication

Accountability fosters transparent communication within the team. This openness ensures that all team members, regardless of their role, are aware of the practice's direction, informed about changes, and aligned with the overarching mission.

Pursuit of Excellence

A culture of accountability aligns with the core value of the pursuit of excellence. Practice owners, team members, and even pet owners become part of a collective journey toward continuous improvement, ensuring that the practice never rests on its laurels but consistently strives for excellence.

Build Your VPOS: Action Steps for Accountability

1. **Take Responsibility for Your Practice**
   Reflect on your personal satisfaction as a practice owner. If there are aspects of the practice that are unfulfilling, stressful, or don't make you happy – take action and change them! This is extremely empowering and can transform your relationship to your practice.

a. Reflect on a few recent problems or mistakes that happened in your practice. For each one, consider how you, as the owner, could have been more accountable and helped prevent that problem, either through better training, resources, facilities, or support.

b. List out at least three things that are happening in your practice right now that you don't like or wish were different. For each of these, write down at least the *first step* you could take in improving that area. Then, take that step as quickly as possible!

2. **Commit Time to Working On Your Practice**

a. Get your calendar and schedule at least one hour per week when you will work *on* your practice.

b. During this time, you will work on addressing issues and opportunities and figuring out how to implement all the other beneficial programs you'll find in this book. If you don't set aside the time to work on this, nothing will ever change.

3. **Establish Regular Meetings**

This will come up many times in future chapters because regular meetings are critical to implementing any programs or initiatives in your hospital. Meetings contribute specifically to accountability because team members know they need to complete specific tasks or commitments and share their progress with the team in the next meeting.

a. Commit to having regular practice meetings. Minimally, you must have a leadership meeting and an all-staff meeting at least once per month. I've included a list of recommended meetings at the end of the next chapter on "Planning."

    b. Schedule your meetings and orient your team on what is expected from them in each meeting.

4. **Track Accountability and Training Progress**

Do you have a training program and accountability for both the trainer/mentor and the trainee?

    a. Establish a systematic approach to track training and tasks and ensure accountability. It doesn't have to be complex. It can be as simple as a notebook or a whiteboard or as sophisticated as a full project management software system. Choose what makes the most sense for your practice – but no matter what, have *somewhere* that critical tasks are tracked as to ownership, status, and date for completion.

    b. Regularly review and update this system during team meetings.

Accountability Is the Best Lifestyle

Being a business owner involves a lot of ups and downs. It can be exhilarating and inspiring one day and exhausting and demoralizing the next. By embracing personal accountability for both the ups and the downs, you empower yourself to take control of your business and shape it in the direction that creates the most fulfillment and success for you and your team while delivering great care for your patients and your community.

It's important to remember your reasons for becoming a practice owner in the first place. I bet that at least one reason you chose to be a business owner is to ensure your practice delivers on the mission of veterinary care in the way that you think is best.

You still have that power – if you use it!

References

1. Novo Melo, P., Martins, A., and Sousa, P.M. The relationship between leadership and accountability: A review and synthesis of the research. Journal of Entrepreneurship Education [Internet]. 2020;23(6). Available from: https://www.abacademies.org/articles/the-relationship-between-leadership-and-accountability-a-review-and-synthesis-of-the-research-9618.html

2. Drake, M. Detox your practice: How to eliminate toxic team members and avoid hiring them [Internet]. DVM. 2022;360. Available from: https://www.dvm360.com/view/detox-your-practice-how-to-eliminate-toxic-team-members-and-avoid-hiring-them

3. Carucci, R. Leaders, stop avoiding hard decisions [Internet]. Harvard Business Review. 2018. Available from: https://hbr.org/2018/04/leaders-stop-avoiding-hard-decisions

4. Kavanaugh, J. and Tarafdar, R. Break down change management into small steps [Internet]. Harvard Business Review. 2021. Available from: https://hbr.org/2021/05/break-down-change-management-into-small-steps

5. Lederhouse C. Study Fair pay, appreciation for work top factors in employee retention. American Veterinary Medical Association [Internet]. www.avma.org. 2024. Available from: https://www.avma.org/news/study-fair-pay-appreciation-work-top-factors-employee-retention

6. Rabasca, R.L. When Leaders Make Mistakes [Internet]. www.shrm.org. 2020. Available from: https://www.shrm.org/topics-tools/news/hr-magazine/leaders-make-mistakes

7. Han, E. How to Create a Culture of Ethics & Accountability in the Workplace [Internet]. Business Insights Blog. Harvard Business School; 2023. Available from: https://online.hbs.edu/blog/post/ethics-and-accountability-in-the-workplace

8. Wickman, G. Traction: Get a Grip on Your Business. BenBella Books, Inc; 2012.

9. Blackout in Southwest leaves 5M in the dark – CBS News [Internet]. www.cbsnews.com. CBS News; 2011. Available

from: https://www.cbsnews.com/news/blackout-in-southwest-leaves-5m-in-the-dark/

10. Okano, K., Kaczmarzyk, J.R., and Gabrieli, J.D.E. Enhancing workplace digital learning by use of the science of learning. Ito E, editor. PLoS One. 2018;13(10):e0206250.

4

Planning

Where are we now?
Where are we going?
And how are we going to get there?

The year I lost my dad was especially tough for me. It was not expected, and I did not get to say goodbye to him. Even as I write this now, I tear up a little. We were very close, and it was a big loss. I was not fully engaged in my practice while I was grieving. However, the structured meetings in the practice continued, and my team picked up the slack that I was leaving. What got us all through this difficult time was adhering to the meeting schedule, my showing up after some grieving time, and all of us collectively pushing through together.

When I give talks to veterinarians, I sometimes get pushback on how much time my team spends in meetings. In reality, it's not very much

---

Veterinary Leadership: A Practical Guide for Practice Owners and Managers, First Edition. Michele Drake.
© 2025 John Wiley & Sons, Inc. Published 2025 by John Wiley & Sons, Inc.

time, though when I review all of our meetings in one talk, it can seem overwhelming. Meetings are essential because they keep everyone on the same page. You never know when this is going to suddenly become more important. If you own a practice long enough, there will be times in your life when you have very little to bring to the planning process for a while. My team helped me through my grief by keeping the show on the road, and they were able to do this because of the plan and the structure we had created together. Having a plan and schedule are important. Stick to them.

As a young veterinarian, the prospect of buying my first practice at the age of 27 was both exhilarating and daunting. I worked tirelessly in the office nearly every day, and it felt like the pace of everything was moving faster than I could keep up with. With just myself and three and a half employees, it might not have been a massive operation, but it was a lot for me to manage.

I quickly realized the importance of stepping back and gaining a broader perspective on my practice. So, every week, I would carve out an hour, escape from the demands of the clinic, and "take myself out for coffee." Armed with nothing more than a pen and paper (yes, I've always been a bit old-school), I'd sit down to reflect, plan, and strategize. This was back in the day when laptops were a luxury and tablets were still in their infancy.

Looking back, it sounds almost quaint, but it was during those solitary coffee breaks that I began to understand the essence of effective planning. There's something powerful about physically putting pen to paper, jotting down ideas, and organizing thoughts. It was a simple act that laid the foundation for the more complex planning strategies I would develop over the years.

My planning sessions weren't only confined to the coffee shop. I also initiated monthly staff meetings, which, at that point, consisted of me and my three key employees gathering at my house. I made sure to sweeten the deal with some good food to keep the atmosphere casual and conducive to brainstorming. It was a humble beginning, but I understood the importance of collaboration and communication in driving our practice forward. I knew I needed their help and buy-in toward what I was trying to accomplish.

Fast forward to today, and my approach to planning has evolved significantly. What started as a basic routine to manage a fledgling business has grown into a sophisticated system of strategic thinking, collaboration, and execution. I've surrounded myself with a talented team, each member bringing unique skills that complement our collective ability to plan, execute, and achieve our goals.

One principle that has remained constant throughout this journey is the importance of asking, *"Where are we now? Where are we going? And how are we going to get there?"* Your team needs to know your vision and support your plans. You cannot do this alone.

Take Yourself out for Coffee (and Perspective)

Whether you're a seasoned veterinarian or a practice manager, the struggles are real. It's sometimes easier for an outsider to see the issues and offer straightforward recommendations; but from within, it may seem like an impossible mountain to climb.

If you're feeling overwhelmed by the challenges within your practice, my advice is to step outside the daily grind. Physically get out of the practice. Take yourself out for coffee. Take a moment to think about what is overwhelming you. Quite often, the exercise of thinking this through outside of the practice is all you need to do to realize you have solutions.

Reflect on why you chose this profession, what drives you, and what your practice stands for. The answers often lie within ourselves, and it's a matter of taking the time to uncover them. I also do this exercise while I'm riding my bike. It's amazing what we can discover when we have some quiet time to think.

Being thoughtful about the direction of your practice is key. It's not just about making decisions; it's about making the *right* decisions. Once you've reflected on your purpose and goals, it's time to engage with your key team members. Share your thoughts on what needs to happen and, more importantly, listen to what they think. In my experience, when it's the right course of action, a consensus often emerges effortlessly.

I'm fortunate to work with a team of 11 other doctors, and despite the diversity in our approaches, we generally find ourselves in agreement. The secret? We're aligned at a fundamental level on our mission, and we know what is ultimately the right thing to do. Part of the "right thing" is that we align on how we practice so that clients and staff get the same messaging from each of us. Finding common ground is not as challenging as it may seem, and fostering open communication is instrumental in achieving it.

Plan for Growth and Adaptation

It's impossible to ignore the profound impact that effective planning has had on both the growth of my practice and the unique lifestyle it affords me. When I first ventured into practice ownership, the demands were relentless. Working six to seven days a week was a necessity, given the small team and myriad responsibilities of being both a practicing DVM and a business owner.

One key philosophy I embraced early on was the idea of *hiring before the need becomes urgent.* I've taken a proactive approach, extending 6–12 months ahead for DVMs and 3 months ahead for other crucial positions. This allowed me to navigate growth without getting into a crisis situation. Anticipate your needs, stay ahead of the curve, and hire accordingly. It's much tougher to make time to hire when you're already underwater. And hiring under pressure can lead to hiring people that aren't right for your business. Always hire ahead of needs.

By aligning hiring decisions with a well-thought-out growth plan,[1] I gained the confidence to expand my team without ever having to let someone go. This foresight was crucial during challenging periods, such as the economic downturn in 2008. While many businesses struggled, we weathered the storm by closely monitoring our financials, adjusting our hiring strategy, and maintaining a laser focus on delivering exceptional care and service.

During that stagnant economic phase, we conducted an internal audit, examining every aspect of our practice. The goal was to understand how consumer behavior was evolving and identify areas where we could enhance our services and create even more value. This introspective approach ensured that we not only sustained our business but also positioned ourselves for future growth.

Discipline in planning and the ability to adapt to changing circumstances have been instrumental in shaping not just the success of my practice but also my personal lifestyle. Through careful planning, I've crafted a career that allows me to thrive professionally while maintaining a balanced and fulfilling life outside the clinic.

Crafting a Comprehensive Plan: Balancing External and Internal Factors

A robust planning process involves a balance between external factors that shape the industry and internal dynamics that govern the everyday workings of a veterinary practice.

First and foremost, I start my day with a cup of coffee and the *WSJ*. This daily ritual, instilled in me since childhood, provides valuable insights into the broader economic landscape, consumer behavior, and global trends. It's also a quiet time when I take a few minutes to think before starting the day. When my children were young, I didn't let this slide – I got up 15 minutes earlier to have this alone time to settle my brain before starting a busy day.

Follow Trends – Don't React to One-Off Issues

A common pitfall I've observed in our profession is allowing a single client's feedback to disproportionately influence our business decisions. Rather than succumbing to this tendency, I focus on identifying trends. For instance, in 2008, it became clear that the advent of handheld devices such as the iPhone was reshaping how people accessed information. I knew nothing about the digital world and didn't own an iPhone in 2008. But it didn't take much brilliance to realize how important this tool would become to daily living. Embracing this change, I sought to understand digital marketing and social media. I could see how they would reshape consumer choices. I sought out people in my network who understood where things were going and asked for their help in shaping a plan for my practice to stay ahead of the curve.

I was a bit worried in 2008 that we were "behind the times" – but as it turned out, we were actually a decade ahead of most other veterinary practices. I still talk to practice owners today in 2024 who are not doing what my practice was doing in 2008 with respect to social media engagement and community building. But it's never too late to look over the situation and make a new plan.

Changes like these also affect employee behavior and needs, and without a plan, you can easily be thrown off by them. The seismic shift triggered by the COVID-19 pandemic was an obvious example, but there have been many other smaller shocks in the business and economic landscape over the 30 years I've been in practice. While our plan may need to be adjusted to deal with changes, we are still vastly better off having a clear plan as a starting point. This keeps us from fumbling blindly when conditions change.

Unlocking the Potential Within: Strategies for Team Empowerment

Planning also involves adapting to changes in technology. Interest in understanding digital transformation has grown steadily in recent years and has led to the increased availability of research and thought leadership on how leaders should approach technology influences in their strategic planning. Current research identifies enabling and disruptive technologies as key drivers for business model innovation (BMI),[2] displaying the need for practice managers to understand new technologies and utilize that understanding to empower and support their teams.

A couple of years ago, we transitioned to a cloud-based PIMS (Practice Information Management System). While the team handled this shift admirably, we faced a new challenge in implementing an online appointment scheduler. Managing two buildings, though they were adjacent, posed a unique hurdle in finding a system that seamlessly integrated with our workflow. This internal struggle highlighted the importance of aligning technological advancements with the practical needs of our practice.

We must also consider the evolution of medical practices, surgical procedures, and internal protocols. Regular team discussions address the efficiency of our surgery patient flow and the effectiveness of client communication during these critical moments. The decision to update policies or introduce new vaccines and medications prompts collaborative conversations on how to implement these changes.

Our leadership meetings tackle these essential aspects head-on. From managing diabetic cases to canine upper respiratory vaccine discussions, we deliberate on how to disseminate this information to our team effectively. It's not just about updating policies, but also about ensuring that every team member is well-versed in the changes. This often involves identifying which segment of our staff needs specific information, sparing them from information overload while equipping them with the essentials.

Empowering our team with knowledge is an ongoing process, one that extends beyond our monthly meetings. Bulletins, such as a recent one addressing the upper respiratory viruses, serve as timely reminders of the importance of aligning our knowledge base. In these communications, we outline both the protocols for managing cases and the rationale behind them. It's about fostering a collective understanding of our goals, procedures, and the reasons behind them.

Nurturing Financial Health: A Prescription for Prosperity

Early in my entrepreneurial journey, a seasoned friend imparted invaluable advice: *"Run your practice as if you might have to sell it within six months."* This perspective not only applies to a potential sale someday, but also serves as a fundamental principle for day-to-day operations.

There's a misconception in this industry that discussing profit is somehow like being a "used car salesman." In my opinion, this is a detrimental mindset. I am driven by a dual commitment: providing stellar care and service while ensuring fair compensation for my team's hard work. To achieve this balance, we have to pay attention to our financials.

Have Budget Milestones and Follow Them

It's vital to have milestones for key components of your financials. The most important are *payroll* and *drugs and supplies*. These are the areas where we have the most control, and together, they account for the majority of the expenses in most hospitals. I'm going to share a few numbers here that I use in my practice, but it's vital to work out the right numbers for your practice, which may be different based on your type of practice, community, types of services, and growth goals, among many other factors. For example, a specialty hospital will likely have numbers that are very different from mine. To make sure you have these figured out correctly for your practice, I highly recommend working with an accountant who specializes in veterinary practices. You should also consider joining VMG, which provides benchmarking to show you how your numbers compare to other similar practices around the country.

Payroll

One very important aspect of financial planning is the meticulous management of payroll. Over the years, I've aimed to keep payroll close to 40%. This percentage, while it's not rigidly fixed, serves as a guidepost, alerting us to potential staffing imbalances. Going above 40% of course means we're overstaffed to some degree, but dipping significantly below 40% is not necessarily good, as it can mean we are shorthanded and need to hire to avoid overworking our employees. This metric guides us in making informed decisions about efficiency improvements or strategic growth to support higher payroll.

If payroll is coming in high, rather than making abrupt staff cuts, our approach involves assessing systems and operations for potential enhancements. It's an evaluation of what we do and how we can do it better; it ensures that our growth aligns with our financial resources. I've had some practice owners chide me that this number is too high, but then others say they are amazed that keeping it this low is even possible. Every practice is different, but everyone must pay attention to this number to ensure the success of the practice. San Diego County, where my hospital is located, is an amazing place to live, but it has recently been called the most unaffordable city in America. This number is based on the cost of gas, food, restaurants, and housing. Every community has a microeconomic environment that must be factored into financial planning.

Drugs and Supplies

I aim to keep my cost for drugs and supplies below 15%. There are many ways you can get more control of these costs. Consider joining a group purchasing organization (GPO) if you're not part of one. These organizations leverage a larger group of practices to negotiate lower prices. Stay in close contact with your distributors and the pharmaceutical companies whose products you use in your hospital. Product lines are constantly evolving, and prices and rebates often change.

In addition to these strategies, one important step I've taken in my practice that helps me keep these costs in line is to ensure alignment among my team on the specific products and protocols we use. I've often visited other veterinary hospitals and seen two or three different parasiticides on the shelf. When I've asked the owners why this is the case, they've told me that doctor A likes this product, doctor B likes that product, and so on. This lack of alignment not only confuses their clients, but also leads to inflated inventory and higher prices for these products. By aligning your team onto one set of products, you increase the amount you're purchasing from that company, and this will generally lower your costs. In subsequent chapters, I'll dig further into the benefits of having your DVMs aligned on products and protocols, but this is one very tangible benefit of that alignment.

While certain factors like rent and mortgages are often beyond our control, the above elements are levers we can pull to optimize our financial health.

Don't Neglect Your Fee Schedules

Another important aspect of financial planning involves fee schedules. With inflation higher than it's been in decades, addressing pricing has become essential. I've seen many practice owners who would rather absorb increased costs for payroll, drugs, and supplies rather than confront the possibility of raising prices. This is not about squeezing more money from clients, but simply asking them to recognize the value we provide. With our focus on exemplary medical care and service, we've never had any real pushback from clients when we have to raise prices. Remember that they've seen the price of everything else go up already, so it's not going to be a big surprise.

There's one specific thing about raising prices that is often overlooked by small business owners. If you don't have a lot of experience reading your profit and loss statements (P&Ls), this may not be obvious, but it's vital to understand: One dollar in increased revenue through gaining a new client is probably worth about 15–20 cents in profit to your practice (depending on your margins). But one dollar in increased revenue through a price increase is a whole dollar in profit to the practice – so it has 5× or more the impact on your bottom line. Again, this doesn't mean you should raise prices indiscriminately, but it does mean you should be attentive to anywhere your pricing is too low and not be afraid to increase it. If you're doing a great job on the other lessons outlined in this book, your clients will be fine with paying a few dollars more for the care you provide.

You Really do Need to Confront Your Financials

I know many practice owners don't feel as comfortable working on a P&L as an IV or an Rx – but it's actually just as important to the health of your practice over the long term. Neglecting financial considerations jeopardizes the foundation of your practice. It impacts not only your ability to attract and retain talent, but also the overall stability and appeal of your clinic to both clients and staff.

Strategic Planning and Proactive Financial Management

While many veterinarians adopt a reactive stance toward their finances, I advocate for a more proactive approach, one that involves setting benchmarks and strategically planning to meet and exceed them.

The key lies in monthly and annual planning sessions. We review our KPIs (key performance indicators) every month. This includes payroll numbers, volume of business, new client numbers, and any other number we may be working on, such as compliance in certain areas. Mid-year, we evaluate where we are in relation to our annual goals. In December, we begin to assess the prior year and use some of this information to help us with our SWOT analysis (Strengths, Weaknesses, Opportunities, and Threats) and goal setting in January. Our January meeting is the time to review the financial and performance data of the prior year, review our SWOT together, and set goals for the new year. This proactive approach sets the stage for intentional financial planning, laying the groundwork for a successful year ahead.

However, as the saying goes, "No plan survives contact with the enemy." The unforeseen challenges, such as the unprecedented wave of the COVID-19 pandemic, underscore the need for adaptability. While our initial plans might have been thrown into disarray, it was our proactive financial management that allowed us to navigate the uncertainties effectively.

Rather than viewing benchmarks as rigid constraints, we regard them as guiding stars, offering direction and insight into the financial health of our practice. Going above the 40% payroll figure is not a crisis; it's a signal. It tells us when to reassess our current staffing needs or if we are over-staffing at certain times. The aim is not merely to cut costs but to recalibrate so we use our resources in the best way possible. During COVID, we had a hard time keeping up with hiring and training. I was asking too much of our staff but I let them know that we were vigorously working on correcting this. Again, we explained where we were with staffing, our planned, current goal, and how we were going to get there. This included building out additional space in the building next door to create an Annex with six more exam rooms. Everyone knew our building was too small for how much we had grown, but we had a plan to handle this, and everyone on the team knew that plan. Either you tell your entire team what is going on or they will begin to make up stories.

Again, you can't overdo it when it comes to sharing your current vision and plans with your team. They need to know to be on board.

Working on the Business vs. Working in the Business

The distinction between working on the business and working in the business can define the course of your professional and personal life. Having witnessed the spectrum from dysfunction to prosperity in various practices, I've come to recognize the importance of being not just a practitioner but a strategic planner toward your own success.

It can be scary to make the transition from practicing DVM to visionary and business owner. I've found that many practice owners back away from this and default to where they are comfortable, which is usually being busy in the exam room or in surgery. By setting aside time each week to work *on* my business, I was able to force myself to become a disciplined business owner. I spent this time on many different issues. Some examples include working on staffing; finding efficiencies; reviewing my P&L; working on our mission statements and culture; and so on.

As the practice grows, the demands increase, but the core principle remains the same: dedicate the time needed for intentional planning and share that journey with the team.

Shape Your Practice, Shape Your Life

A practice owner's life varies. Some find themselves ensnared in a cycle of exhaustion, stress, and financial strain, while others – like the mentor I had the privilege of working with – demonstrate that it is possible to live a balanced and fulfilling lifestyle.

As I reflect on those early days, I recall observing a practice owner who seemed to have "cracked the code" to a life well-lived. A seasoned businessman with a penchant for strategic planning, he orchestrated a practice that not only thrived in terms of medical excellence, but also provided him with the time and freedom to savor life beyond the clinic walls.

I wondered, "What set him apart? What were the elements contributing to his fulfilling lifestyle, and how did that impact the overall dynamics of the practice?" There were unmistakable characteristics that I observed, which helped me in developing my own approach.

One crucial element was a commitment to planning. The practice had a dedicated Practice Manager, and regular meetings were held to discuss various aspects of the clinic's functioning. This deliberate approach to business planning, a practice I would later adopt in my own clinics, laid the foundation for a well-organized and high-functioning environment. Within this discussion of planning, I'd be remiss if I didn't stress the importance of financial planning once again, as, whether you realize it or not, your practice's financial goals and your personal financial goals are closely linked. Organization within your personal finances can influence your practice's financial performance and vice versa[3] – and planning lies at the heart of both.

The impact of this approach became evident when the practice owner began taking time off. This departure from the stereotypical image of the overworked and continually stressed practice owner was a revelation. It was proof that a well-structured practice, underpinned by thoughtful planning, could foster not only professional success but personal fulfillment as well.

Witnessing this healthier and happier work environment left an impression on me. It was a stark contrast to what I had seen in dysfunctional practices, where chaos reigned and employees were caught in a cycle of stress. While I may not have consciously analyzed every detail at that time, the contrast between these environments undoubtedly played a role in shaping my approach to practice ownership.

I grew up in a family that ate breakfast and dinner together almost every night. I was committed to doing this with my family, as well. Learning how to plan was vital to achieving this personally important goal.

In sharing this experience, my intent is not to paint a utopian picture, but to challenge the prevailing narrative that associates practice ownership with misery and exhaustion. There is an alternative path – one where strategic planning, a supportive team, and a commitment to a balanced life come together to create a practice that thrives on all fronts.

Bring Discipline to Your Planning

Maintaining consistency in planning requires discipline and accountability. It's acknowledging that, no matter how busy the practice becomes, the regular meetings and planning sessions are non-negotiable. Let go of the excuse of "I'm too busy." Recognize that an hour a week and possibly a few longer monthly meetings would be time well spent in planning and that this is not a luxury but a necessity if you're going to build the practice you really want.

Unite Your Team Through Planning

One of the most powerful benefits of consistent planning is the creation of alignment within the team. When everyone is involved, informed, and engaged in the planning process, a sense of shared ownership emerges. Team members no longer feel like passive participants; instead, they become architects of the practice's journey.

Missed meetings, on the rare occasion they occur, serve as reminders of the value derived from consistent planning. The need to reconvene becomes apparent when there's a sense of loose ends or when it becomes evident that alignment is a bit adrift.

When your team is united through planning and well-synced, taking the "baby steps" needed to launch new projects or initiatives becomes far easier to facilitate. Some of the projects you may want to tackle, such as creating a better culture or implementing a new technology, may seem daunting. There will be times in your career when you can barely keep your head above water, and you may be tempted to put off all planning. This is a mistake. If you're short a DVM or if you've lost a key staff member, it can feel catastrophic. During these times, continue to meet, plan, and just take "baby steps" toward these goals. This will keep your goals at the top of your mind, and it will force you to reconsider your plans and maybe find someone else on the team who can run with the project for a while. If you do not meet and at least discuss the projects, goals, and issues, then absolutely nothing will change or progress. Remember: Baby steps are better than no steps at all.

Strategic Tools for Effective Business Management

The amount of structure you need in your plans can vary based on the situation. Historically, we had been a bit more casual about some aspects of planning. However, during COVID, the very fast-paced changes in how we did business, and the massive increase in volume and staffing required a more disciplined approach. This is where the Traction system I described earlier came into play.

I had read *Traction: Get a Grip on Your Business* years before, and I reread it as COVID started. I had my entire leadership team read it, as well as *The Five Dysfunctions of a Team*. We immediately utilized the lessons from these books to launch the Traction system as the overarching structure for our leadership team meetings and as a better format for accountability and keeping up with all the changes.

Our monthly leadership team meetings evolved to span six to eight hours, a concentrated period allowing for a deep dive into critical issues. The team, comprising six key individuals, found this format to be immensely effective.

The Traction system introduced several key components[4] that significantly enhanced our business management:

1. **Rocks for the Team:** Identifying three key objectives ("rocks") for the entire team to accomplish in the next quarter provided a clear roadmap for collective success.
2. **Individual Rocks:** Assigning specific tasks or goals to each team member ensured accountability and focused efforts on individual responsibilities.
3. **Commitment and Scheduling:** Before concluding each meeting, team members committed to specific tasks, creating a tangible action plan. In addition, scheduling the next three monthly meetings well in advance ensured ongoing commitment and participation.
4. **Succinct and Organized Meetings:** Emphasizing preparation, the team compiled notes from the previous meeting, updated on individual accountabilities, and streamlined discussions to ensure that meetings were succinct, well-run, and organized.

People don't mind being in meetings when they are organized, succinct, and purposeful. If you're getting pushback from your team on participating in meetings, look for how you can make them feel as effective and engaging as possible. The steps above are a great start.

One final note on meetings: I never have pharmaceutical reps come in and speak to my staff. When there is a new drug available, our DVMs get briefed with video, conference, or Zooms from the pharma company, and then our doctors present to the team how we plan to use and support this new medication.

The Power of Planning

Having a solid plan for your practice can benefit you, your team, and your community.

Elevated Team Morale

Planning not only ensures the smooth operation of your practice but also fosters a supportive and collegial environment. When team members have a forum where they can share concerns, discuss challenges, and collaboratively solve problems, the workplace becomes a space where stress is managed collectively. This elevated team morale is a key component in combating the mental health crisis prevalent in the industry.

Effective Crisis Management

Planning equips your team with the tools and systems to manage unexpected events or crises efficiently. Whether it's a medical emergency or a negative online review, a well-aligned team that has a clear plan for addressing issues ensures that the practice remains resilient in the face of challenges.

Enhanced Client Experience

Proactive planning makes your practice feel systematic, orderly, and predictable. Clients and their pets appreciate a well-coordinated and efficient environment.

Increased Accessibility and Availability

By planning ahead and hiring staff before the need fully arises, practices can avoid frantic "on-fire" scenarios. This ensures more time for serving clients, taking in clients who couldn't get an appointment elsewhere, or even offering extended hours for critical care.

Reduced Stress

Planning alleviates stress for the owner, the staff, and your clientele. The payoff is not only in business success, but in the well-being of the teams, the satisfaction of clients, and the optimal care of their pets.

Build Your **VPOS: Action Steps for Planning**

1. **Change Your Environment**
   - Identify a location outside your practice and home where you can conduct planning sessions.
     - Find a space that you feel enhances your focus and creativity.
     - Schedule your next planning meeting in this new location. Take the time just for yourself, especially if you have a small practice, or include key members of your leadership team.
2. **Conduct a Comprehensive SWOT Analysis**
   Look over your business and note down a few examples for each of the categories below. As you'll see, these can get very deep and detailed, but you'll want to focus on the areas where you can see immediate ways to take action on an issue. Repeat this at least once a year.
   - *Strengths:* What is working well? What are you great at? What do you do in your practice that sets you apart from competitors?
   - *Weaknesses:* What is not working well in the practice? Where are you having difficulties or challenges with your team, space, or processes?
   - *Opportunities:* Are you fully using all your tools, resources, and systems to reach new and existing clients? Are you training your staff in all the basics of compliance? Are there ways you could better align your team? Are your marketing, website, and social media doing enough to connect you to your community?
   - *Threats:* Are there new competitors in the area? Are there corporate practices coming in that could take market share? How are we responding to new competitors like Chewy? How will we respond to

the erosion of the VCPR that is being driven by new
telemedicine platforms?

3. **Utilize Planning Exercises**
   - Choose one of the items you noted down in your SWOT
     analysis that you're ready to do something about. It's
     often easiest to start with a weakness to fix or an oppor-
     tunity to start pursuing.
   - For this item, write out a simple plan for how it can get
     done. This should include:
     - The goal of making this change
     - Who will be in charge of implementing this plan
     - Deadline for when it should be completed
     - As best you can, write down all the steps needed to
       complete this plan
     - Now, do the first step!

The goal here is not to fix everything that's wrong with your
practice overnight, but rather to create a system and get you into
the habit of creating a plan and executing it. Consistency is the key.
Of course, things will come up that throw you off your plan – but if
you have a plan and you have meetings scheduled to check up on
that plan, then you have something in place that will help you get
back on track.

Remember, these exercises are not just about business; they
shape your pathway to a more balanced, fulfilling, and successful
life as a practice owner.

Bonus Resource: Meetings at The Drake Center

- Leadership Meeting
  - Frequency: Monthly
  - Attendees: Team 1 (Leadership Team)

- Location: Off-site
- Length: Six to eight hours
- Agenda includes: Major plans and "rocks"; changes in protocols or policies; progress toward our annual goals (see details below)
- Staff Meeting
  - Frequency: Monthly
  - Attendees: All Staff (required to attend unless in school, on approved PTO, or sick)
  - Location: In practice or Zoom (with cameras on!)
    - Practice is closed during this time (7:30–9 a.m.)
  - Length: 1½ hours
  - Agenda includes: Highly curated meeting with multiple staff contributing (see details below)
- Pulse Meeting
  - Frequency: Monthly at a minimum – more often during times of rapid change – for example, we met weekly during COVID to manage all the changes in training, compliance, and recruitment
  - Attendees: Team Leads that contribute to the "pulse" of the practice, along with me and the practice manager
  - Location: Zoom (with cameras on)
  - Length: One hour
  - Agenda includes: We ask the team to bring us their perceptions of team progress, how new employees are developing, training information, and any situations or concerns that need to be addressed
- Doctors' Meeting
  - Frequency: Monthly
  - Attendees: Owner and all DVMs
  - Location: Off-site
  - Length: Two to three hours

- Agenda includes: Review CE notes from recently attended meetings; review new drugs and consider using them; ensure our practices and recommendations are aligned so that clients and staff have a consistent experience and messaging regardless of which DVM they are interacting with; create camaraderie and support for the DVMs – this is a meeting they enjoy and look forward to!
- Owner/Practice Manager Meetings
  - Frequency: Ad hoc meeting – can be 1–3 times per month
  - Attendees: Owner and Practice Manager
  - Location: Can be in-house, lunch meeting, or Zoom
  - Length: One hour
  - Agenda includes: Checking in on progress and any issues that come up. This meeting agenda is different every time, responding to the latest developments
- Marketing Meetings
  - Frequency: Monthly
  - Attendees: Owner, Practice Manager, Marketing/Media Coordinator, and/or outside marketing team
  - Location: Zoom
  - Length: One hour
  - Agenda includes: Marketing strategy, upcoming events, promotions, social media, recruitment, website management, and anything else related to connecting our practice with our community
- DEA Meeting
  - Frequency: Monthly
  - Attendees: DVM, purchasing manager, RVT
  - Location: In practice
  - Length: One hour
  - Agenda includes: Reviewing bookkeeping, doctors' licenses, compliance, drug storage, safety

- Drugs and Supplies Meeting
  - Frequency: Monthly or as needed
  - Attendees: One of our DVMs, practice manager, purchasing manager
  - Location: In practice
  - Length: One hour
  - Agenda includes: Reviewing inventory and upcoming needs, pricing strategies, group buying opportunities, and any changes proposed to our standard protocols. Creating accountability for the budget and supply levels, and keeping the team in the loop on any changes

If you think this is a lot of meetings, you're right! I didn't do all of these in the beginning when we were smaller, but as we grew, we needed more coordination to ensure we could maintain alignment with a larger team.

The larger your practice grows, the more time you will need to spend "working on the practice" and this includes meetings. Well-informed and aligned team members work together more productively and effectively, and this more than makes up for the time spent in meetings.

Of course, you will want to create a schedule that works best for your practice, but this is the meeting structure that has been very successful for us.

Leadership Team Meeting Agenda

A week before the meeting, we are prompted to review our lists and update them for all attendees. Attendees are also asked to let us know if they have any items to add to the issues list for group discussion. Then, a week before the leadership meeting, we have a separate pre-meeting with the floor manager team, who may add more items for leadership to discuss.

1. **Icebreaker** – Meetings always begin with an icebreaker or vulnerability exercise. These exercises take about ten minutes, and everyone will answer the same question to keep the conversation on topic. It is very important to begin each meeting with this exercise, and the range of conversation can be truly impressive: Sometimes, they are hilarious, and other times, they are quite somber.

2. **KPIs** – KPIs and numbers we are following or focusing on include payroll, cost of goods (COGS), year-over-year (YOY) review, numbers of exams, fill rates for DVM schedules, tech visits, total new visits and new clients, and number of no-shows. We compare each of the numbers month-over-month and year-over-year to get a complete picture of our performance. We will also often add compliance items that are current goals to the discussion, e.g., taking annual lab work from 60% to 70%.

3. **Staffing Numbers** – We regularly discuss if our staffing needs are being met, if we need to hire, or if staff members need to be moved between departments.

4. **Rocks** – We then move to review the three rocks for the quarter. Discussion is initiated by the primary person responsible for each rock, e.g., new online scheduling system, development of new kennel team protocols, etc. Everyone gets an update and an opportunity to discuss, and the person who owns this rock may ask for help or suggestions. Discussion may or may not follow, depending on the rock and its current status. Quarterly rocks are created depending on the time of year for discussion.

5. **Action Items** – Next, we go through each person's to-do list from the last meeting, and they say "done," "not done," "in progress," or "need help." If they need help, or if a discussion starts, we stop and put this on the "issues list." We have a scribe who uses a whiteboard to create the issues list as we start the meeting so we can make sure we don't miss anything.

6. **Issues List** – To go through the issues list, we present an issue or opportunity, engage in group discussion, find consensus, and then hand out a new action item if needed or move on to the next issue.

7. **Staff Development** – We discuss staff development at every meeting. If "stay interviews" were done, we discuss the interview and decide how to proceed. We review accumulated information on the training progress of newer team members, including mentors' notes, DVM input on skill levels, and new team members' input on where support may be needed.

8. **Flow and Staffing** – We always discussed flow and staffing as an issue, just in general terms, to ensure the entire team is on the same page.

9. **Review Action Items** – We discuss the new to-do lists for each member of the leadership team, including what items may be delegated or communicated to others on the team.

10. **Schedule** – Finally, we review the next two to three months' meeting dates to make sure all are on the same page and all can attend.

11. **Follow-up** – After the meeting, each team member has three days to email the group their to-do list.

Staff Meeting Agenda

I could write an entire chapter on our staff meetings, but suffice it to say that a fair amount of thought and preparation goes into the meeting – not by just one person but by the team. Only one person prepares the meeting agenda, but they can delegate topics to others.

As our staff grew over the years from 4 people to 55–60, the level of prep and types of discussions have evolved a lot. The fact that this is a very important time for the entire staff to be present together warrants a high level of thought and preparation. This meeting has great value. You want to utilize this time well by focusing on topics that are necessary, being very clear with your communication, and inspiring your team. We require all staff to be present for every staff meeting once a month (approximately 10 meetings a year). Since COVID and because of our size, we now do half of our meetings on Zoom and the other half in person. Everyone must be on camera when on Zoom, as this ensures they will be more engaged.

1. **Housekeeping** – We start by covering specific information that we want to make sure everyone is on the same page about, including new protocols, new pricing, new policies, or old policies that need updating or reminding.
2. **Staffing** – The "Staffing" portion of our meeting involves personal introductions of new team members, positions, and mentors. We also use this time to announce changes in staff positions, training plans, etc.
3. **Education for All Teams** – This section is led by the DVMs. This includes things such as new diabetic monitoring devices and protocols, flea and tick education, product updates, and behavior education. Generally, we have two doctors, each spending about 7–10 minutes on each topic.

4. **State of Union** – We utilize this time to discuss where we are now, where we are going, and how we are going to get there. This is done by the practice owner, or a leader who can share new or current vision and plans. This portion of the meeting should be kept brief – 5–10 minutes.

5. **Kudos** – During our meetings, we acknowledge three to four staff members because of how they reflected our culture or supported our mission in their actions this month.

6. **Culture and Values** – Here, a leadership team member may give a brief review of one of the tenets of our culture or one of our core values and the why behind them.

7. **Breakouts** – We like to end our meetings with breakouts of teams for the last 30 minutes for specific education or updates or policies concerning each specific team, e.g., front staff, kennel team, surgery team, or exam room team. This section is organized and planned ahead of time.

This is the general layout of each meeting, which lasts one hour if done over Zoom or an hour and a half when done in person. We always have food, and, of course, everyone is paid for their time.

References

1. Drake, M. Growing a veterinary practice: Insights from The Drake Center for Veterinary Care. wwwdvm360com [Internet]. 2023;54(8):70. Available from: https://www.dvm360.com/view/growing-a-veterinary-practice-insights-from-the-drake-center-for-veterinary-care

2. Vaska, S., Massaro, M., Bagarotto, E.M., and Dal Mas, F. The digital transformation of business model innovation: A structured literature

review. Frontiers in Psychology [Internet]. 2021;11. Available from: https://www.frontiersin.org/articles/10.3389/fpsyg.2020.539363/full

3. Felsted, K. and Saunders, M. Make it happen: Personal and practice financial growth for veterinarians. Vetted [Internet]. 2020;115(8). Available from: https://www.dvm360.com/view/make-it-happen-personal-and-practice-financial-growth-for-veterinarians

4. Wickman, G. Traction: Get a Grip on Your Business. BenBella Books, Inc; 2012.

5

Culture

> Either you decide what you want your culture to be, or someone
> else will decide for you – and you may not like the outcome.
> Not defining your culture is not an option.

*I fired my first employee less than three months after buying my first
hospital. It was extremely difficult. There were only three and a half
employees, and she was our only RVT. She had been with the hospital
for five years. However, I realized that she was consistently not nice to
our veterinary assistant and our kennel employee. I did not think I had
the skill set to teach someone how to be nice. So I fired her and began the
search for a new RVT. I explained to the few staff why I fired her and that
I would always insist on a team that is kind and respectful to each other.
That day, the kennel employee said to me before she went home, "Ding
Dong the witch is dead." From that point on, they knew I had their backs*

Veterinary Leadership: A Practical Guide for Practice Owners and Managers,
First Edition. Michele Drake.
© 2025 John Wiley & Sons, Inc. Published 2025 by John Wiley & Sons, Inc.

and would not allow people to be mean in our practice. This was the beginning of a very strong culture in The Drake Center. Firing people is hard, but if you want to have a specific culture and someone is disrupting that culture, either they need to change or they need to go. Anything else will leave your hospital in a constant state of distrust and create continual stress for your team.

Exactly What Is "Practice Culture?"

The dictionary defines "culture" as *the ideas, customs, and social behavior of a particular people or society.* Organizational culture builds on this understanding of culture and has been defined as "a feeling of pride, fellowship, and common loyalty shared by the members of a particular group."[1]

In the context of veterinary practice, I like to define culture more personally as *how we play in our sandbox.* It's about how team members interact, collaborate, and uphold the values and mission of the practice. It's about how we handle stressful situations and extremely busy days requiring triage strategies, and how we bring a high level of communication to accomplish these tasks. It's about how we hire and train. It's about feeling good about what we accomplished and thanking each other at the end of the day.

How Culture Relates to Your Mission

I define the *mission* of a veterinary hospital as *the purpose we have every day.* It's what we do as a business. The *culture* would be *how we behave while accomplishing this mission.*

Mission and Culture at The Drake Center

At The Drake Center, our mission is *to provide the best medicine and surgery in a compassionate environment for our patients and unsurpassed customer service for our clients.*

Our culture is that *we work together with kindness, respect, teamwork, and fun.*

In my three decades as a practice owner, I've encountered thousands of my peers grappling with various challenges in their veterinary practices. Time and again, the root of many struggles can be traced back to the practice culture. While people cite many reasons for business difficulties – from economic factors to staffing woes – a failing or misaligned culture often underpins these issues.

Culture is the heartbeat of any veterinary practice. It drives every interaction, decision, and outcome within your business. When the culture is positive, uplifting, and aligned with your vision, it becomes a powerful catalyst for success. Employees are motivated, clients feel valued, and most importantly, the level of care provided to our animal patients reaches its highest potential.[2]

Conversely, a failing culture can be a practice's undoing. In such environments, nothing seems to work right. Communication falters, morale dips, and the quality of service inevitably suffers. This often leads to a vicious cycle of employee turnover, client dissatisfaction, and business stagnation.

Embracing a positive and aligned culture isn't just about creating a pleasant workplace. It's about unlocking the full potential of your practice. It's about building a team that shares your passion, vision, and commitment to excellence. When culture is prioritized and nurtured, the possibilities for what your practice can achieve are limitless.

Why Culture Matters

A strong culture is intimately connected to trust. Our ability to work quickly and effectively in challenging circumstances depends on the ability to trust the competence, good intentions, and reliability of our teammates.

When trust is strong, team members assume positive intentions on the part of their teammates, and they give them the benefit of the doubt when small, inevitable mistakes happen. We make better decisions, deliver better patient care, and achieve better business outcomes.

When trust is low, team members think the worst of each other, assume deceptive or covert intentions in one another, and second-guess their teammates. They tend to catastrophize or exaggerate their fellow employees' mistakes, which causes people to slow down and focus on "CYA" rather than delivering great patient care and service.

I met a doctor once who explained to me that she kept catching her team lying to her. I was really perplexed by this, as I cannot even imagine thinking that about my staff. I believe there must be a significant lack of trust in this practice. I can't imagine how this practice owner can get through the day wondering if her team is telling her the truth. I honestly think the cultural problems in this practice probably stemmed from the owner's own distrust of her staff. This would have to change to begin building a strong team.

Culture Is a Daily Activity

Every member of our team, from the top leader to the newest recruit, knows exactly what to expect in the behavior of the team when they step into our practice each day. This level of predictability and alignment isn't just about routine but rather a shared commitment to our mission. It reduces the stress of coming to work when you know how people are going to behave. Everyone on the team appreciates this.

Contrasting our culture with some I've observed elsewhere, the biggest difference is that we truly live our culture every day. Our cultural values aren't just a poster on the wall in the breakroom. They are integral in who we hire (and fire), how we train our team, and how we work with our clients.

We have a zero-tolerance policy for bad behavior that's not aligned with our culture. We don't aim to be authoritarian. Instead, we focus on setting a clear and strong example of what is acceptable and what is not. This has created a culture that naturally deflects people who don't align with our values while powerfully attracting people who will be a great fit.

When you walk into The Drake Center, the strength of our culture is immediately palpable. It's positive, mission-aligned, and focused. We don't allow individuals, whether they are doctors, technicians, or even clients, to derail us from our mission. Our strong, positive culture is appreciated, respected, and actively upheld by our team. In addition, since we have a strong culture, it is obvious if we've made a bad hire – the team lets us know.

Walking the Talk: Upholding Core Values in the Face of Challenges

It's vital as a practice owner that you "walk the walk" and not just "talk the talk," especially when it comes to protecting and upholding your culture. The owner and manager must actively display the culture they want to create in their daily behaviors and management.

I recall one incident that particularly exemplifies this commitment. A technician, who had been with us for three years, overstepped the bounds of acceptable behavior in a dramatic and unacceptable way. This employee had a disagreement with another team member and chose to express it by cursing at the person in front of other staff members. This was not just a breach of professional conduct; it was a violation of the ethos of our practice. When people behave badly, it's very disruptive to the flow of care and service. This behavior was a direct threat to our mission, creating unnecessary distractions and a negative environment.

I wasn't present when the incident occurred, but I was informed about it by one of my doctors, who asked her to leave immediately.

The next morning, I fired this employee. This action was not about punishment, but about protecting our culture and reinforcing the message that certain behaviors are simply not tolerated. This was a clear message to all our employees: We are committed to providing you with a good place to work. I believe it is the responsibility of owners and managers to provide a healthy workplace for their team. Healthy people appreciate this.

The employee in question was generally a good worker but had shown a tendency to need more ego validation than others. We had managed to work with her up until this point, coaching her on smaller issues. However, this outburst was a clear line-crossing moment. It was important for me to show that our commitment to a positive, professional environment was not just words, but would be backed up with action.

In dealing with the aftermath, we focused on coaching and supporting the other employees involved in the incident, emphasizing that while disagreements may occur, the way we handle them matters. Our culture is about more than just avoiding conflict; it's about handling it in a way that is constructive and aligned with our values. This incident was a powerful reminder to everyone at The Drake Center that our culture is something we live by every day, in every interaction.

Laying the Foundations for a Positive Practice Culture

For practices that may be struggling with their current culture, it can be difficult to know where to start. My advice to owners and managers is to sit down outside of the practice[3] and have an open-hearted discussion about the status of the culture as it is now. Allow your team members to be vulnerable and honest about how they're feeling in the practice.

Next, discuss how you would like your culture to be. *What vision do we have of a great culture? What do we need to do to get there?*

There will be no change if the owner, manager, or any other key personnel are not involved in this initial discussion.

Once you have your core team, sit down, discuss, and plan. Start small, with a few key individuals, and then gradually expand the circle. The key leadership must be 100% aligned before beginning the discussion with the entire team.

Culture change doesn't happen overnight. It requires patience, commitment, and a clear vision. As you progress, invite more people who are interested in fostering a positive culture to join the effort and then begin to invite the larger team into this process. Eventually, you will include the entire team because everyone must participate and buy into the process of having a great place to work.

Remember, it's not about making a grand announcement and expecting immediate change. It's a gradual process that requires engagement, dedication, and a clear understanding of the desired direction. Working collaboratively and being supported by others in the practice makes this journey less daunting and more achievable. The goal is to shift from a culture that might currently be suboptimal to one that everyone is excited to be a part of.

The Transformative Effect of Positive Culture on Recruitment and Growth

Hiring during COVID was difficult but not impossible. We sought doctors who were not just professionally capable, but also aligned with our culture – positive, communicative, and team-oriented. We were able to hire four additional doctors during COVID because our own team recruited like-minded doctors for the practice, and we have a very strong reputation for providing a healthy, supportive workplace. In addition, we needed to hire many support staff for these new doctors. There were very few applicants who already had the needed skills. In my experience, the local support staff who are regularly hopping from practice to practice are generally not good culture fits for our team. Instead, we hire for culture fit, attitude, and desire to learn, and then we train for skill.

In our team meetings, the positive and collaborative spirit is palpable. Everyone, from the kennel lead to the practice manager, is committed to supporting each other. Recently, a kennel lead said they needed help due to the influx of new recruits. Together, the team made a plan and immediately rallied to assist. This proactive and supportive attitude is a testament to our culture and how it facilitates our operational efficiency and growth.

Our approach to recruitment and hiring, heavily influenced by our culture, has made my manager's job easier. We don't just look for employees; we look for team members who will thrive in and contribute to our positive and dynamic environment. My practice manager, Chris, does a great job in the interviewing process of getting people talking with open-ended questions and recognizing signs of good or bad culture fit. Other veterinary practice owners have taken a similar approach to assessing culture fit and the similarities – or differences – in personal and practice ethics early on in the interview process, and have reported smoother hiring experiences for everyone involved, as well as reduced instances of ethics exhaustion.[4]

We have a lot of young 20-somethings, who may be in community college or just graduated from Davis or UCLA, and are considering veterinary school. These are great employees, but they need training. They fit our culture because they are good communicators, they have a strong desire to work for us and learn, and they are good team players. Because we have a large influx of young people without specific skills, training is constant. Our team knows that this can be hard on the long-term team members, but because they are highly aligned with our culture, they recognize the value of training new team members well so they can deliver on our mission.

In our practice at The Drake Center, we integrate continuous training into our culture. Professional growth and development are planned for everyone on the team several times a year. Obviously, some are more driven than others, and we parcel out the plans accordingly. The team embraces this continuous learning environment without fuss, which is integral to our success. This approach is a key factor in attracting new team members, setting us apart from other veterinary hospitals.

We also take great pride in our website, which we are constantly improving. Our website is a true reflection of who we are, and I believe this transparency is what draws applicants to us. They get a sense of our culture, our commitment to care, and our community involvement right from the start. This online presence, coupled with our strong reputation in the community as a top-notch veterinary hospital, naturally attracts talent. We frequently see young people from the local area applying to join our team, who are the children of long-time clients.

Our reputation extends beyond our immediate locality throughout San Diego and beyond. For example, we recently had an extern from UC Davis, a well-respected veterinary school, who was struck by the positive and distinct culture at our practice compared to her university. I recently interviewed an upcoming graduate of veterinary school who said he wanted to move to San Diego and, after talking to some people whom he knew in the area and looking at our robust website, he asked for an interview.

We rarely place help-wanted ads. In fact, I can only think of twice in 30 years that we have had to advertise for a veterinarian. Regardless, we have only ever had an open spot for a veterinarian for a short period when we've decided to wait for the right person.

Our reputation for having a supportive and well-aligned team also extends to specialists in the area. They often recommend their interns and other professionals to explore opportunities with us, knowing the positive and collegial environment they will encounter. Our own employees are our ambassadors, further expanding our reach in attracting top veterinary talent.

The Power of Culture in Creating Workplace Satisfaction (or Dissatisfaction)

One recent telling story about the impact of our culture at The Drake Center involves a veterinarian, Dr. Lee, who joined us from a corporate hospital in Pasadena. When she first visited us, she was adamant that she wasn't looking to change jobs right away. However, her visit to our center completely changed her perspective ... within one hour.

Dr. Lee's experience in her previous role had left her feeling disillusioned. She was seeking not just a job, but a workplace where she felt supported, valued, and part of a positive team. Her visit to The Drake Center was eye-opening. Within just an hour of experiencing our environment and interacting with our team, she made a decisive choice to join us. This decision wasn't taken lightly; she even made sure to give her previous employer a month's notice, reflecting her professional integrity.

The move for Dr. Lee meant relocating from Pasadena, leaving her familiar surroundings and family. Yet, she felt that the supportive and nurturing environment at The Drake Center was worth this significant change. Her experience shows the profound effect a positive workplace culture can have on individuals. It's not just about the tasks they perform or the salary they receive; it's about how they feel, how they're treated, and the values they share with their teammates.

Dr. Lee's story is one among many that highlight how a positive, supportive culture can not only attract top talent but also deeply influence their career choices and job satisfaction. This narrative underscores the significance of culture in creating a workplace where employees don't just come to work but come to thrive. We have many employees at The Drake Center who have been with us for more than 15 years, and we have zero attrition of doctors. This is a testament to the culture we've created in the practice, and it has a lot to do with our stability and financial success as well as personal development.

I am constantly hearing from practice owners that they are struggling with recruitment. While it can seem like the answer is to hire a recruiter or buy more job ads, often the first and most important step is to work on the culture of the practice, and make it a place people want to be a part of.

Culture and Getting Things Done

Culture is not just about maintaining a happy workplace. It's about having a unified approach toward growth and improvements. Having a strong culture makes it substantially easier to enact new systems, achieve growth, and meet your goals.

Unity and shared vision make it possible to accomplish tasks and implement changes that would otherwise be daunting. A strong culture is the driving force behind your ability to get things done effectively and efficiently in the practice.

Unity Creates Strength

In our practice at The Drake Center, the culture we've nurtured plays a pivotal role in how we handle challenging days.

We've all had those days when you arrive at the practice and a key employee has called in sick, there are two urgent cases plus surgery drop-offs all landing at the same time, and you just know *this is gonna be a tough day.*

On days like these, when the pressure is immense and the workload seems insurmountable, the strength of our team and our culture sees us through. Our entire team, from the doctors to the technicians, the front staff, and the kennel team, pulled together. There is a palpable sense of unity and commitment. Everyone steps up, not just to get the job done, but to ensure that every patient receives the best possible care.

At the end of such a grueling day, instead of feeling drained and worn out, there is a sense of accomplishment and pride. The team high-fives each other, acknowledging the hard work and exceptional care provided.

In many other practices, days like these can be soul-sucking, leaving staff exhausted and demoralized, especially if the team isn't aligned or working cohesively.

Of course, we aim to ensure that such demanding days are not a regular occurrence, as we prioritize supporting our staff and maintaining a sustainable workload. But on those days that do test our limits, our culture of teamwork and mutual support turns challenges into opportunities for us to shine and reaffirm our commitment to excellence in veterinary care.

What Does It All Mean for You? Empowering Practice Owners Through Culture

Establishing a great culture in my practice has been instrumental in allowing me freedom and flexibility that are rare in the world of veterinary practice ownership. I don't need to be present at the practice for it to stay positive and on-mission. Initially, my participation in establishing the culture was vital, but now the culture is so deeply ingrained in our doctors and key staff that it thrives regardless of who is on for the day. We have a strong leadership team embodying our culture, which provides the framework for alignment and managing all issues and opportunities. When the team knows your mission and culture, they know how to handle any situation.

When I'm at the practice, I'm just another part of our culture. When I'm not there, the culture and team function the same way. This consistency is the result of years of nurturing and adhering to our mission and culture. Challenges and new situations still arise, but my team is well-equipped to handle them. Everyone contributes their input, and decisions are made based on our collective understanding of who we are and how we approach problems.

This is not to say that I am not an important part of the team, but rather that the team does not rely on my presence to function effectively. A key component to this is having a competent and culturally aligned hospital manager. This role is critical as they handle hiring, employee relations, and other integral aspects of the practice. My manager and I work closely together, ensuring that our vision and approach are aligned; when we find we're not aligned, we engage in constructive dialogue to find a common ground. She challenges me to make good decisions.

In essence, the culture at The Drake Center doesn't just create a better working environment for the staff; it also provides a more sustainable and fulfilling role for me as the practice owner. It's the assurance that the practice not only survives but thrives, even in my absence, that makes all the effort to build and maintain this culture truly worthwhile.

At the end of the day, building a strong practice culture takes work. But it's more than worth the effort. Here are some of the most significant benefits of investing in your practice culture:

Increased Operational Efficiency

A positive culture fosters a high-functioning team, enabling the practice to handle more cases effectively and to grow.

Enhanced Recruitment and Retention

A strong culture attracts more applicants and retains staff longer, reducing the need for and expense of recruitment efforts.

Improved Autonomy for the Practice Owner

A well-established culture allows the owner to step away from day-to-day operations without compromising the practice's functioning or ethos.

Reduced Workplace Stress

A positive culture significantly reduces stress, benefiting both staff and the owner and leading to a healthier work environment.

Stronger Team Resilience in Challenging Times

During difficult periods, a cohesive culture enables the team to handle increased workloads and stress more effectively.

Heightened Employee Engagement and Productivity

Employees in a positive culture are more engaged and productive, leading to better client service, improved business outcomes, and more development of each staff member.

Competitive Advantage in the Industry

A strong culture differentiates the practice in a competitive market, making it more appealing to both clients and potential employees.

Reduced Turnover

A robust culture within a veterinary practice leads to significant retention. When staff members feel valued and are part of a nurturing environment, they are less likely to leave.[5] This stability fosters expertise and continuity in patient care, reducing the strain and costs that most practices are experiencing from frequent hiring.

Enhanced Job Satisfaction

A positive practice culture elevates job satisfaction. Staff members who find meaning and camaraderie in their work are more engaged and productive. This satisfaction transcends the professional realm, contributing to overall well-being and life satisfaction.[6]

Diminished Mental Anguish

In cohesive teams, mental stress is alleviated. When individuals know they have the support and understanding of their team, it reduces the sense of isolation and mental burden, especially in challenging situations. A supportive culture acts as a buffer against the high-pressure environment of veterinary practice.

Adaptive and Responsive Teams

A well-aligned team can adapt to changing situations with agility. In practices where team members can confidently step into different roles as needed, there is a fluidity and efficiency that enhances overall performance and patient care.

Palpable Atmosphere Difference

The atmosphere in a practice with a strong, positive culture is noticeably different. This palpable change creates a more welcoming environment for clients and a more enjoyable workplace for employees, enhancing the reputation of the practice.

Improved Patient Care

The cornerstone of any veterinary practice is patient care, which is invariably heightened in a practice with a unified team. Each member contributes effectively, ensuring comprehensive care and attention to each patient.

Building a Better Industry Reputation

As positive cultures become more prevalent, the veterinary indus-try's reputation as a desirable and fulfilling field of work is bolstered. This reputation can attract new talent and retain existing profes-sionals, addressing the industry's workforce challenges.

The prevailing culture within veterinary practices has implica-tions not only for the quality of care provided, but also for the well-being of those who dedicate their lives to this wonderful profession. Unfortunately, the industry is grappling with the pervasive problem of poor workplace cultures. I believe that a significant portion of the workplace woes in veterinary medicine, such as burnout and anxiety, are substantially reduced in a healthy workplace. Healthy people want to belong to a practice that is well managed. If we pro-vide this, they will come.

Adopting a strong, positive culture in veterinary practices isn't just about improving one clinic; it's about uplifting an entire profes-sion, enhancing care quality, and creating a more sustainable and fulfilling work environment.

Build Your VPOS: Action Steps for Your Culture

Reflect on Your Role as an Owner

- Watch Dr. Drake's short video on culture at www.geniusvets. com/culture
- Start by introspecting on your core values, the reasons you started your practice, and your vision for the future. Write this down so you can refer to it later. Questions to ponder:
  - What motivated me to start this practice?
  - What type of "sandbox" do I want for myself and my employees? What type of impact will this have on us?

- Is there anything I'm doing that could be a roadblock to a better culture?
- What are my current practice culture, mission, and values?
- What is my vision for my culture and values?

Engage Key Team Members
- **Leveraging Team Strengths: You need your team to buy into and add to your vision of a great culture. Let them know you really want to provide a good place to work and you need everyone to make that happen.** Identify and collaborate with team members who positively embody the practice's values. Their strengths are vital in shaping and reinforcing a positive culture. Questions to ponder:
  - Who are the positive role models in my team?
  - How can I utilize these team members' strengths to improve the overall culture?
  - What are the current barriers to open communication in my practice?
  - How can we create an environment where team members feel comfortable sharing their thoughts?
- Set up a meeting with your key team members to discuss their perspectives on practice culture.
  - Openly discuss where your practice culture is now and where you want it to go.
  - Discuss any barriers and how to overcome them. It is usually one or two people in the practice who have negatively affected the practice. Can you bring them into the discussion of how you want to change the culture and how you need their help?
  - Document your decisions about the culture in writing so they can be shared with your broader team.

Bring the Plan to Your Broader Team

- Once you've worked with key leadership to create a written statement of your desired culture, bring this to a staff meeting and announce it.
- Invite discussion and feedback so that you can get buy-in from the team.

Address Naysayers

- Address individuals resistant to change constructively, understand their concerns, and make decisions about their fit in the future practice.
- Engage in honest dialogue with those who are resistant to the new cultural rules.
- Develop a plan to integrate them or to remove them from the team if necessary.
- Be firm in your plans to progress to a better culture. Coach people as much as possible, but in the end, you must let go of any employee who is not willing to move forward with the practice plan to improve culture.

Conduct Regular Check-Ins

- Regularly assess the progress of cultural initiatives through your leadership meetings and staff meetings.

Celebrate Small Wins

Acknowledging and celebrating even small achievements that align with cultural goals can significantly motivate the team. For example, at The Drake Center, we have a program called "Kudos." I reach out to all the DVMs and key staff and ask them to name anyone who has shown exceptional performance in following our culture and core values; then, we recognize that person in a staff meeting, thank them, and buy them lunch. We also have a "treasure chest" where anyone can give

Kudos to another team member, who then gets to pull a prize out of the treasure chest, such as a $10 gift card for coffee or food:

- Identify and publicly acknowledge small victories.
- Give recognition to employees who display your desired culture. Be specific.
- Organize events or activities to celebrate these successes.

The Path to a Positive Practice Culture

Building a great culture requires dedication and effort, but the rewards are immeasurable. In my own practice and with numerous successful practices nationwide that I've had the opportunity to work with, the benefits of a thriving culture are clear: improved team morale, higher employee retention, better client satisfaction, and, most importantly, enhanced care for our beloved patients.

The steps outlined in this section are not just theoretical concepts; they are practical, actionable strategies that have been proven to yield results. This might seem daunting at first, but remember, every significant change starts with small, consistent steps. The journey to reshaping your practice's culture into one that is vibrant, supportive, and successful is indeed challenging, but it is also deeply rewarding.

By committing to this path, not only do you pave the way for a more harmonious workplace, but you also contribute to the greater good of the veterinary profession. The ripple effect of a positive culture extends beyond the walls of your practice, influencing the broader industry and elevating the standards of veterinary care. Embrace this journey with optimism and a positive attitude, and watch as your practice transforms into a place where both people and pets thrive – and an inspiration to other practices to do the same.

References

1. Fukami, C., Hutton, B., Hoffman, D., and Garcia, R. Understanding the Impact of Organizational Culture in Veterinary Practices. American Animal Hospital Association; 2016.
2. Drake, M. Culture 101: creating a healthy practice environment. wwwdvm360com [Internet]. 2024;54(12):46–6. Available from: https://www.dvm360.com/view/culture-101-creating-a-healthy-practice-environment
3. Drake, M. Stepping outside of the practice is critical for improving it [Internet]. DVM. 2022;360. Available from: https://www.dvm360.com/view/stepping-outside-of-the-practice-is-critical-for-improving-it
4. Dennis, S. Swipe left to get it right: avoiding ethics exhaustion by matching with the right veterinary team [Internet]. DVM. 2018;360. Available from: https://www.dvm360.com/view/swipe-left-get-it-right-avoiding-ethics-exhaustion-matching-with-right-veterinary-team
5. STAY, PLEASE A Challenge to the Veterinary Profession to Improve Employee Retention [Internet]. aaha.org. American Animal Hospital Association; 2023. Available from: https://www.aaha.org/practice-resources/research-center/white-paper-form-the-path-to-increasing-retention-in-veterinary-medicine/
6. The Link Between Healthy Workplace Culture and Optimal Personal Wellbeing AAHA CULTURE ROUNDTABLE [Internet]. American Animal Hospital Association; Available from: https://www.aaha.org/globalassets/04-practice-resources/practice-culture/aaha_culture_roundtable.pdf

6

Focus

Run your practice as if you might have to sell it in six months. That level of focus will make you a success, regardless of whether or not you ever decide to sell.

There are so many things going on in your practice as a DVM. To be good doctors, we need to focus all of our attention on listening to our clients and then focusing on our patients. Listening well and being present with our patients as we examine them is crucial to good care. While we are performing our duties as veterinarians and working with our teams, we will see small issues (and maybe some big ones) that need our attention as owners.

New practice owners need to take the time to focus on these issues away from the practice; otherwise, our thoughts will be interrupted. It took me a few months of working six days a week as a DVM to realize

Veterinary Leadership: A Practical Guide for Practice Owners and Managers,
First Edition. Michele Drake.
© 2025 John Wiley & Sons, Inc. Published 2025 by John Wiley & Sons, Inc.

that I would also need to spend some time thinking and planning to move the practice in the direction I wanted it to go.

Mentorship Is Vital

Knowing what we don't know and seeking help in these areas is vital to success. Early on, I was smart enough to hire a veterinary accounting firm to do my bookkeeping for me. Monthly accounting reports are essential to running a good business, and having the support of true accounting professionals allowed me to focus on the other aspects of practice ownership that I excelled in.

However, looking back, one of the most beneficial outcomes of my relationship with the accounting firm was the connections I gained through them. The firm introduced me to a veterinarian who was retiring and might be able to help mentor me.

We instantly connected, and our relationship evolved into one of mutual respect and friendship. He was more than just a veterinarian; he was a good businessman with a wealth of experience that I was eager to tap into. His only goal was to help me be a strong practice owner.

Our meetings were infrequent, a couple of times a year, but each session was transformative. He looked over my financial records, taught me how to review them monthly, and offered practical advice, such as how to adjust fees and manage payroll more efficiently. His philosophy was simple yet profound: *Run your practice as if you might have to sell it in six months.* This approach meant a more disciplined and focused approach to all aspects of running a business. There is an urgency to get things right if you might have to sell in six months.

Though I didn't always implement every suggestion, I valued his insights. They were my homework, challenges to overcome, and opportunities to grow. His direction went beyond the numbers; he taught me to be flexible and adaptive as a leader, to be attuned to the ever-changing dynamics of a small business, and to make decisions in a timely manner. He said he watched so many practice owners who were unable to make decisions and move forward, which strangled their ability to have a great practice.

As our friendship endured over the years, so did my admiration for his business acumen. He continued to make waves in the veterinary world, working with corporations like Pfizer and building large veterinary and pet care facilities. His journey underscored the importance of being more than just a veterinarian; it was about being a visionary in the field and sharing your experience and wisdom with others.

This mentorship was my lifeline in those formative years. I delved into veterinary business literature, seeking wisdom and strategies to elevate my practice. Yet, I soon realized that not all the advice in the industry resonated with my vision. As we've discussed throughout the previous chapters, vetting information and finding sources that are accurate, reliable, and driven by results and experience is crucial in this profession. Just because an article appears in *Veterinary Economics* does not mean it is sound advice. I learned to trust my instincts, drawing insights from a variety of sources, including mainstream business journals like the *Wall Street Journal*.

As practice owners, we need not just to learn about new drugs and skills, but also remain adept at thoughtful leadership and business practices.

The Results of Not Focusing on Your Business

Often, veterinarians work incredibly hard but find themselves in a frustrating loop of financial struggle, being dissatisfied with their staff, and at odds with clients over financial matters. Most veterinarians are much more comfortable in the exam room or surgery suite than they are in managing their businesses, and they use the excuse that they are "too busy" to focus on their business. But in reality, we must take control of our own destiny, or we are just reacting.

As we established in Chapter 4, planning is at the heart of focusing on your business. Planning ahead and taking the time to focus on what's next for your practice equips you with the knowledge, data, and process know-how needed to make crucial decisions for better practice management. Take managing staff schedules and payroll, for example. Both are essential aspects of practice management, but when practice owners spend more time in the exam room than in observing what support your practice needs, trouble isn't far off. Always hire before you are in serious need because it takes time to hire and train the right person. This approach of prioritizing focus and planning has allowed me to manage my practice efficiently, not overwork our team, and keep that critical payroll number in order.

When COVID-19 struck, this underlying issue became more pronounced. Many veterinarians, already overwhelmed and financially strained, reached their breaking point. While some were forced to reduce services and consolidate staff,[1] some chose to reduce their practice hours or even sell their practices as a way to cope with the stress and workload.

They shifted to a lifestyle-focused model, reducing hours and enjoying more personal time, which indeed brought more happiness to many teams.

However, the question that often gets overlooked is: what does the community need? While it's essential not to overwork the team, the solution isn't necessarily to cut back on services but rather to expand the team thoughtfully. By hiring and training new people, a practice can meet the needs of its community without overburdening the existing staff. Rising to the challenge of growth allows us so much more flexibility for our staff and also allows us to provide a higher level of care and service. As we grew, this allowed more flexibility for myself and my team for our lifestyle choices. We have 11 doctors and 55 staff now, and this gives us a lot of flexibility. This is awesome for personal and family choices. Something to consider: The same people who tell me they don't want to grow are the ones who also wish they had more flexibility for their team and themselves.

Isn't This Too Capitalist? "I'm Not in it for the Money"

None of us got into veterinary medicine for the money. I bought my first practice early in my career because I was passionate about care and service, and I decided to put my money and time where my mouth was. Being conscientious about making sure your practice is financially stable and profitable is not about greed; it's about responsibility and sustainability. Running a healthy business translates into a healthy team, great care, service, and profitability, which allows us to reinvest in what matters to us and creates options for lifestyle and family decisions.

Running a veterinary practice is about more than just caring for animals. It involves ensuring that your staff is paid adequately, bills are covered, and the business is not perpetually stressed by financial constraints. Ignoring the importance of profitability often translates into an environment where standards slip and staff members are unhappy; ultimately, the quality of animal care suffers.

The mindset of always being ready for a potential sale isn't about a relentless pursuit of profit. It's about maintaining high standards, being prepared for any eventuality, and ensuring the long-term health and success of the practice. This approach benefits everyone involved – the team, the clients, and the business itself.

Focus and Clutter – Managing Your Space

In my journey of purchasing and running three veterinary hospitals, I've observed a common theme: *clutter*. Most veterinary hospitals that I visit are cluttered, and statistics suggest that this isn't just a veterinary industry problem, but, rather, a wider organizational issue that many businesses fall victim to. In a survey of 2,000 office workers in the United Kingdom, 40% of respondents admitted that an untidy workspace inhibits their productivity,[2] also likely affecting their ability to focus on their core tasks. Research has shown a relationship between the presence of clutter within a work environment and an increased likelihood of emotional exhaustion, stress,[3] and reduced productivity. But, clutter isn't just physical; it clogs the mind and obscures your vision. To me, clutter represents more than just disarray and signifies a lack of focus, often becoming a barrier to seeing what's essential.

Every night, I make it a point to clear my space. A clean counter, devoid of distractions, is crucial for me to start the next day fresh. This might seem trivial, but it's symbolic of larger principles in business and life: clarity and focus.

In my experience, a cluttered environment often reflects a cluttered business approach. If a practice is visually chaotic, it often indicates a deeper issue with how the business is managed. Is there a clear vision? Is this vision well communicated to the team? Is the mission obvious? Is the culture palpable every day?

A clean and organized space is more than just an aesthetic choice. It's a reflection of how you run your business. It's about maintaining focus and having the mental clarity to make informed decisions. This approach, while seemingly simple, has profound implications for the health and profitability of a veterinary practice. In addition, by taking care of the hospital and keeping it clean and decluttered, you are showing respect for the place of business and the people who work there.

In the end, managing your space effectively is directly connected to managing your business effectively. It's about prioritizing and decluttering not just your counters, but also your business processes and strategies. And that's how, in my view, you build a valuable veterinary practice.

Focus Makes You More Successful in a Competitive Environment

After I acquired The Drake Center, a nearby hospital run by a veteran veterinarian suddenly closed for a week, posting a "Gone Fishing" sign on their door. This abrupt closure led many of their clients to our facility, which was then quite modest in size. These clients, accustomed to a very different level of care, were astounded by the quality of service we provided. It was a revelation for many, as they expressed their surprise at the standard of veterinary care we offered.

I remember feeling a mix of pride and compassion, assuring these new clients that they should return to their previous vet when he came back, and we would send records. However, many opted to stay with us, attracted by the higher quality of care we provided. As one client said, "We had no idea that a veterinary office could be like this."

The other veterinarian, who had been in business for 30 years without significant growth, resented our expansion and our focus on hiring more doctors to meet growing demands. Of course, we continued to focus on our mission, and this helped us grow to the size we are today.

Build Your VPOS: Action Steps for Focus

Make Sure You Have a Mission, Core Values, and a Defined Culture
If you don't, start there. "Know thyself."

Make a Commitment to Look at All Aspects of Your Business in a Disciplined Manner
This includes finance, cash flow, marketing, leadership, payroll, HR issues, and training.

Focus on the Financial Health of Your Practice

- Determine if you have the right bookkeeper in place.
  - Does your current bookkeeper work with other veterinary practices?
  - Do they fully understand the cash flows and accounting issues for your business?
  - If so, great! If not, consider finding a bookkeeper who has this experience.
- In collaboration with your bookkeeper, set some goals for the financial well-being of your practice. A competent bookkeeper/CPA will lead this discussion and help push you where you need to improve.
- If you do not have a standing meeting with your bookkeeper to review your monthly financials, put this in place and get it done ASAP.
- Review your financials for the past month. Compare your key numbers to industry benchmarks for payroll, drugs and supplies, and overhead.
  - For any categories that are off target, make a quick action plan to get them under control.
  - A whole book could be written just on this topic, but truly, the most important step is to *look* at your numbers monthly, and when they're out of whack, make a simple plan to improve them. This isn't rocket science, just discipline and consistency. A good bookkeeper and CPA, especially one who knows our industry, is a treasure. Find the right one.

Stay Informed About Industry Trends

Keeping up with industry trends is essential for adapting and growing your practice. Understanding national and local trends can provide insights into how to shape your business strategies.

- Read several veterinary journals and online newsletters a month.
  - Write down at least three important trends you found and, for each of them, write down at least one way you could adjust your practice to better align with that trend.
- Set aside a specific time each week to review these materials and take the above step of looking for relevant trends.
- Ensure that your key practice leaders also do the same and set aside this time for reflection and analysis of the changing industry.
- Consider joining a veterinary business group such as VMG or TVC. Peer consultation and accountability can be very motivating.

By following these exercises, you can take concrete steps toward improving your business focus and operational efficiency. This will put you in the best possible position regardless of your "exit strategy" for your practice. Maybe you'll continue to own it for many years and never want to sell. But by running your business like you might have to sell it, you will be running the strongest business possible and maximizing your options for the future.

References

1. Howard, B. Veterinary practice in a pandemic: six experiences [Internet]. VIN News Service. 2020. Available from: https://news.vin.com/default.aspx?pid=210&Id=9623465&f5=1

2. Study Reveals The Impact of Messy Desks | Blog [Internet]. Brother, UK. 2017. Available from: https://www.brother.co.uk/business-solutions/insights-hub/blog/business/2017/workplace-study-reveals-the-impact-of-messy-desks

3. Dao, T. Office Clutter and Its Influence: Assessing Engagement, Satisfaction, Tension, Stress, and Emotional Exhaustion [Internet]. DePaul University; 2019. p. 47. Available from: https://via.library.depaul.edu/cgi/viewcontent.cgi?article=1322&context=csh_etd

7

Teamwork

> Your team cannot read your mind. They need to hear what you're thinking and how they can be involved.
> Everyone wants to be a part of something great.

It's been a long time since I was just starting out as a new practice owner, but I have surprisingly clear pictures in my mind of my team coming to my house in the evening for our staff meetings in my little apartment in Encinitas, California. I would order pizza and salad, and we would sit around my table and go through a very basic agenda. I knew early on that, in order for me to accomplish anything, I needed their support, buy-in, and input to anything I wanted to accomplish.

Your team cannot read your mind. They need to hear what you're thinking, and how they can be involved. Everyone wants to be a part of something great. I wanted and needed their help to honor our mission and

Veterinary Leadership: A Practical Guide for Practice Owners and Managers,
First Edition. Michele Drake.
© 2025 John Wiley & Sons, Inc. Published 2025 by John Wiley & Sons, Inc.

become a great veterinary hospital. Taking the time to connect with your team brings so much value to your work environment and your goals. Build a team and work together.

Teamwork Is Always Essential, But Especially During Tough Times

The chaos and uncertainty of the COVID-19 pandemic was a test for leadership in every practice. I remember waiting for the *WSJ* to be delivered to my house in the morning; then I would turn on national and local news to get updates from the California governor and the federal government as well. In addition, I had many emails, Zooms, and impromptu meetings with my leadership and the entire team about the ever-changing reality we were living in. It was a tough time as a leader, but it was also a time for us to put on our big girl/boy pants and lead our teams.

Times of challenge are actually a great time to more fully connect with your team. Let them know you have a plan and that together, you will weather whatever is thrown at you. I'm proud of how our team stepped up and worked together during those times.

I remember distinctly how calm our practice actually was during those early days, considering the circumstances. We emphasized caution where needed and maintained our focus on the mission of our hospital. We dealt with the changing masking and PPE guidelines and inconsistent direction from certifying authorities. We reworked our client communications to facilitate curbside service and payment methods, and deployed a text automation platform that we repurposed from the hospitality industry (we were their first veterinary client), and used it to reduce our egregious phone call volume.

Our commitment to providing exceptional care and service became a grounding force amidst the chaos engulfing the world. While others panicked, our team found solace in the routine of coming to work and focusing on what we do best. I reassured my team that this virus was unpleasant but was a very low risk for healthy young individuals. The media often encouraged people to panic. As a doctor, I felt as qualified as anyone to read the actual medical information and share it with my team in a consistent and calm manner. We put on our PPE, adapted to the change in business flow, and continued to provide excellent care.

Maintaining normalcy was no easy feat. But unlike stories I heard from colleagues whose teams dwindled due to factors ranging from fear to enhanced unemployment benefits, The Drake Center did not lose team members during that time. In fact, we only had two employees who needed to stay home for their health, and we accommodated them with phones at home and access to our Practice Information Management System (PIMS). They were a great help even from home.

I recall a friend who managed a major hospital on the East Coast, sharing how most doctors decided to stay home, citing issues with childcare or other challenges. I do know that his hospital struggled with chronic poor morale and culture issues before COVID. The decision for all of the docs to stay home during a time when the hospital and clients needed them demonstrated a complete breakdown of supporting the mission of the hospital and the team who needed them. No doubt, some readers will be up in arms with my lack of sympathy for the doctors at this hospital. However, as a practice owner who raised two kids myself during my career, I believe there were solutions for childcare if people wanted to find them. While we cherish our family-centered approach at my practice, we also recognized that it was vital to find solutions because our patients and clients needed us. And frankly, none of us really wanted to be sitting at home. We believed in the mission, and that belief fueled our determination to keep our doors open. We worked as a team to find solutions and be creative to stay completely staffed the entire time through COVID.

A corporate practice down the street from us closed up entirely because they just couldn't deal with the complexities of staying open. Of course, their clients needed somewhere to go, and many of them found their way to The Drake Center. My mantra during that time became, "We'll get them in. If someone needs their pet to be seen, we'll figure out how to see them. Our community needs us." One client said she had called five hospitals in our area before she called us, and we were the only practice willing to see her pet that day. She was so very happy with our care and service.

We ultimately grew substantially during COVID. And I'm also happy to say that the practice has sustained that growth and has not shrunk back down as many practices have done post-pandemic. In fact, we continued to see significant growth into 2023. I believe that our commitment to teamwork and a shared sense of mission were critical to this accomplishment.

Building a Strong Foundation: Team Structures

Now, let's dive into one of the most important drivers of The Drake Center's success: our well-defined team structures. Structured teams that understand their roles and how they contribute to the achievement of company goals have been found to be more well coordinated and more effective, especially for teams with greater longevity.[1]

Starting with just myself and just a few employees, our leadership team initially encompassed the entire staff. A leadership meeting and a staff meeting were the same thing. However, as we grew, the leadership team became a compact group of four to six people.

Team One: The Leadership Team

In any hospital with five or more employees, it's crucial to have a leadership team consisting of representatives from the front staff and the back staff, as well as the manager and the owner. This minimum of four people forms the core group responsible for coordinating efforts and ensuring alignment across all aspects of the practice. If that is your entire staff, then that is your leadership team. I grew steadily from one doctor to 11 over 30 years. Our leadership team, as well as the amount of time spent managing the practice, evolved to meet the new challenges and opportunities that came with this growth. We refer to this leadership team as "Team One."

The key to this structure's effectiveness lies in the dedication and loyalty of each team member to Team One. In the book, *The Five Dysfunctions of a Team*, Patrick M. Lencioni[2] stresses the importance of Team One members being completely loyal to each other. Disagreements are not only okay, but actually encouraged within that team *while they are figuring out their plans.* However, once decisions are made, it's critical that all members of Team One support each other and the decision that has been made. This unity allows Team One to present a consistent and aligned front to the rest of the team, which then creates teamwork across the organization.

Team Collaboration

In the earlier chapter on "Planning," I've described the types and frequency of our meetings and the structure of these meetings. This chapter will focus on the leadership team and how we make decisions. The key to a well-functioning team lies in:

1. Starting with *open discussion*;
2. Coming to *clear agreements*, and documenting them in writing; and
3. And then each team member giving *full support* to the decision once it's made.

Andy Grove, the CEO of Intel who helped guide that company to over $20 billion in revenue, outlined these principles in his great book, *High Output Management*.[3]

The beauty of this model is that it encourages open discourse without the fear of dissenting opinions but, at the same time, it requires that, before we move forward, Team One is fully aligned, and everyone knows what is being agreed to.

Clear agreement is the linchpin that keeps the team on the same page. It's not just about having a discussion; it's about reaching a consensus that is documented, ensuring everyone understands the path forward. This is especially important once we are back in the practice with the broader team. Everyone on the team should get the same answer from Team One if they ask a question about a new plan. This proactive approach minimizes confusion and fosters collective responsibility.

Mandatories Are Vital in Creating a Cohesive Team

While your business should never be rigid, there are certain issues where strong alignment across the team is vital for patient care and client service. I've found that mandatories are essential for maintaining a cohesive and effective team.

Having a set of non-negotiable rules in the practice doesn't mean you need to dictate every decision from the top down. Instead, it's about establishing guidelines that create a framework for collaboration. I've never had to resort to a rigid "my way or the highway" approach. Good decisions, more often than not, emerge from collaborative discussions where everyone's input is valued.

Collaboration isn't about eliminating any differences of opinion; it's about navigating them with respect and consideration. Any team will face occasional disagreements, especially when it comes to policy and medical care decisions. However, these differences should become opportunities for growth rather than points of contention.

For instance, deciding on a standardized approach to certain treatments might spark discussions among your doctors. When this happens in my practice, I encourage team members to express their preferences, and we find solutions that accommodate everyone's concerns. It's about striking a balance between individual perspectives and delivering on our overall mission.

With that said, once you go through the discussion process and arrive at a standardized protocol, you should feel very comfortable simply requiring that all team members abide by it. This creates consistency in care and predictability for your clients. Clearly communicated and well-thought-out mandatories can define the "edges of the highway," keeping your team all moving down the road together rather than wandering off.

The Ripple Effect of Disarray

I've spoken to many practice owners who feel uncomfortable requiring their associates to do procedures in a specific way or standardizing choices of medications for flea and tick or heartworm prevention. These doctors may feel that "everyone should do it their way" or that they "don't want to be dictators." But they don't realize that this inconsistency actually slows the practice down, creates inefficiency, is very tough on the staff, and confuses pet owners.

For clients to entrust us with the care of their beloved pets, there must be a consensus within our team.

Imagine if a pet owner visits your hospital three different times, sees three different doctors of veterinary medicines (DVMs), and has three different medications recommended for the same condition. This is confusing, and it degrades the service. It's also the best way to lose the trust of clients. *Which of your doctors should they believe?*

Or imagine if you're a tech helping to prep for surgery, but you have to prep for it three different ways depending on which DVM is doing the surgery. This is a recipe for stress, mistakes, and burnout, all of which reduce the quality of care.

In my experience, disarray within a team can have a demoralizing and disengaging impact.

By embracing the process of "open communication, clear agreement, full support," we avoid the harms caused by inconsistent operations. Our decisions become the compass guiding us, and team members rally behind these choices, knowing they contribute to a cohesive and effective practice.

Dr. Peter Weinstein advocates for systems and processes in veterinary management that lead to consistency[4] and repeatable outcomes for both staff and clients. Optimally chosen team members, with the support of clear and direct processes, are a recipe for success and can help eliminate the negative ripples of disarray within a practice or clinic environment.

Our approach to teamwork is a part of our culture. When we hire a new DVM, we have them visit and interview, spend one or two days in the practice, and have a social outing with the doctors. Our culture is very important to us, so we only hire DVMs who want this type of team experience in their workplace. I also make it clear that we work as a team, we build consensus on how we practice, and then we all abide by that consensus.

This team-focused mindset among all of our doctors allows us to have open and productive conversations on how we deliver care to our patients and what tools and techniques we utilize or recommend. An example of this would be the new monoclonal antibodies. They are a great addition. At our monthly DVM meeting, we educate ourselves (most of us have Zoomed with the rep prior to our DVM discussion), and we agree on how we plan to market and utilize these products and what kind of follow-up we would all use. This way, front staff and techs can have a clear message, so they can best support the clients and the practice with clear communication.

Years ago, we were approached by some Merck executives who were intrigued by the exceptional utilization of their product, Sentinel, in our practice. Their curiosity led to a deeper exploration of our methods. They couldn't figure out why we used so much more

Sentinel than other practices. In fact, at that time, we were only a five-doctor practice, but we were told we were the biggest seller of Sentinel in San Diego (by a large margin). It turned out that the answer was simple: We had evaluated all the potential products, realized Sentinel was the best fit for our clients, and recommended it 100% of the time unless there was a special reason to do otherwise. We trained all of our staff on the flea cycle and why we recommend this product, and we made consistent recommendations.

In most practices, the pharmaceutical reps told us, the norm was a diverse array of doctors choosing their preferred flea-and-tick medications. The consequence? A disjointed front desk and exam room experience, where clients received conflicting information from different team members. We stood out by presenting a unified front with a clear message.

As a side note, while it's not the only reason we do this, having aligned recommendations for products will reduce your inventory costs and improve cash flow. It will also make you very popular with your distributors and pharmaceutical reps, who will then work harder to take care of your practice.

Merck asked if I would speak to other hospitals about how to align recommendations and keep a smaller selection in their pharmacies as well. In one particular hospital, I was told before my talk that one doctor would be the "eye-roller" in the meeting and that she does whatever she wants, but the owner does not approach her because she is such a high producer. After asking more questions, I found out that this doctor basically had her own little "practice within the practice," which she ran however she wanted to. This created a terrible culture where the rest of the doctors and team felt very disrespected by her behavior. This practice also had a massive turnover rate in DVMs. I wonder why.

Whether it's recommending advanced dentistry or explaining the nuances of a specialized medical procedure, alignment within the team streamlines the communication process. Clients faced with complicated and sometimes costly decisions are more likely to trust our recommendations when they perceive a cohesive, knowledgeable team.

Navigating Educational Conversations

Educating clients about new products requires time and effort, as we learned with Sentinel, for example. It isn't merely an insecticide; it's an *insect growth regulator*. An adulticide was added as needed. This nuanced information needed to be effectively conveyed not only by doctors, but also by the entire team. Education and alignment ensured that everyone, from the front desk staff to the technicians, conveyed a consistent and accurate message.

Maintaining Alignment

Maintaining team alignment is not a "one-and-done" task; it's a commitment to continuous improvement. This will involve regular meetings, collaborative refinements, and a dedication to addressing challenges one step at a time. The investment you make in creating this team alignment pays dividends in the form of enhanced client outcomes and greater trust and understanding among your staff, among many other benefits.

If you ever want to know what type of recommendations are really being made by your staff, use a call tracking system and listen to at least two calls from each receptionist per month. You may want to sit down while you do this, as it can be a bit traumatic! That being said, you can use this as an opportunity to find out what additional training is needed by the front staff. This is not a time to get upset with your front desk. It's a time to bolster your training plans and empower your staff with the correct information. It's also very important for accountability for new hires and their training. Your team members really do want to give clients the correct information, and they need your help to learn this information.

The Seven-Times Rule

As our team has grown over the years, so has the need for effective communication and a continuous effort toward maintaining alignment. I have what I call the "seven-times rule" adapted from the marketing principle[5] of "The Rule of Seven": *An average team member needs to be exposed to new information at least seven times before it becomes ingrained in their understanding.*

In a veterinary setting, where lack of understanding can lead to disasters, this rule becomes particularly vital. From time to time, one of my doctors would throw their hands in the air and say, "How did they make that mistake? We just went over this." My response would be, "Yes, but that was only the third time they heard it." Not everyone needs to hear things seven times, but some do. The way to propagate good information is to have a team that is ready to help new and younger staff members by kindly reminding them of the correct information and not becoming frustrated in the process. This is another reason we included *kindness* and *respect* among our cultural values.

Once you understand the seven-times rule, you can see how vital it is that you have clear agreements among your leadership team on the important messages in practice. Imagine the confusion that results when, instead of hearing the same message over and over, your team is constantly hearing *different* messages. This confuses the team and undermines their self-confidence and trust. Take the time to get real alignment among your leadership and get their commitment to give a consistent message for the team. This will ensure that your team is able to train new staff in a timely fashion, as well as absorb and implement changes in protocols or treatments.

Trust Is the Currency of Alignment

When team members consistently hear the same message from all corners, trust in the decision-making process solidifies. In veterinary medicine, where each case is to some degree unique, our doctors are, of course, expected to bring their own best judgment and decision-making skills. However, when it comes to over-arching decisions that impact the entire practice, alignment is non-negotiable.

In *First Things First*, Stephen Covey[6] explained that you cannot share your vision with your team too many times. It's easy to make the mistake of thinking that your staff knows what's in your head. They do not. I give a talk at almost every staff meeting to remind the team where we are, where we're going, and how we're going to get there; I call this my "State of the Union." I cannot overstate the importance of this concept.

Veterinary medicine is continually evolving. Diseases change, treatments advance, and protocols are updated. Take diabetes man-agement, for instance – a subject that has seen significant changes during my years in practice. It requires ongoing education and alignment within the team to ensure that everyone is on the same page regarding the latest developments. The use of technology has changed how we communicate with our clients tremendously. Regularly sharing the "why" and the "how" with our teams is so very important. This type of communication is a constant presence in a well-run practice. Having systems in place to share communication is imperative.

Nurturing a Collaborative Team Structure

From the early days of my career, I recognized the intrinsic value of inclusive decision-making. Leadership, for me, includes tapping into the collective wisdom of your team.

Your front desk staff, for instance, may have perspectives you might not have considered, such as questions clients might pose or concerns that wouldn't occur to you as a DVM. By involving your front staff in the decision-making process, you can gain valuable insights that will shape better decisions. In addition, getting them involved will increase alignment and buy-in, as well as fostering a collaborative spirit.

Building Strength Through Conflict Resolution

During COVID, as I discussed earlier, I introduced my leadership team to *Traction* and *The Five Dysfunctions of a Team*, which became the foundation of our strategy for maintaining a healthy organization.

The first step involved each member of our leadership team reading the designated books. We utilized a sort of book club discussion of both of these books but actually put into place a sort of Traction system for the operation of our leadership team. This shared learning experience laid the groundwork for our collective understanding of the principles we sought to implement. Armed with insights about process and prioritization from *Traction* and a deeper comprehension of team dynamics from *The Five Dysfunctions of a Team*, we were ready to embark on practical application.

The leadership exercises marked the beginning of a continuous journey of improvement. It wasn't a one-time fix, but a commitment to ongoing development. The exercises became a regular feature of our leadership meetings, addressing specific areas identified for enhancement. Each session was an opportunity for the team to refine their collaborative skills and fortify the foundations of our leadership structure.

The Five Dysfunctions recommends an "icebreaker" at the beginning of each meeting.[2] My partner, Dr. Boehme, is better at this type of leadership than I am, so she leads these at each meeting. It may sound a tad superfluous, but it has truly become an extremely important way to level the playing field and help us all allow ourselves to open up and be vulnerable, which vastly improves the collaboration, effectiveness, and enjoyment of participation on the team.

Team Structure, Communication, and the Art of Adaptation

With the expansion of our practice, we recognized the necessity for a multilayered leadership and communication approach. I've discussed Team One earlier, which is our leadership team. We also designated Team Two, the junior leadership, who then bring information to the broader team. This created channels for information to flow seamlessly between the leadership team and the broader Drake Center community. This multilayered structure allows for more nuanced communication, ensuring that everyone is kept well-informed.

Tiered Team Structure Example

Team One – Senior Leadership
- **Meeting Schedule:** Meets monthly off-site for six to eight hours
- **Purpose:** Deal with all issues and opportunities in a structured manner
- **Who Is Included:** Owner, manager, at least one representative from each sub-team (front staff, back staff, kennel, etc.)

Team Two – Junior Leadership
- **Purpose:** To communicate to the leadership team any issues with staff, schedules, equipment, policy, etc.
- **Roles:** Responsible for helping with training, flow of the hospital, communication with the rest of the staff, upholding policies
- **Who Is Included:** People who have been with the hospital for two or more years and firmly believe in our culture and mission; could include, e.g., floor managers, lead kennel attendants, and receptionists

The Flow of Information Is a Two-Way Street

Team Two, while not directly part of the leadership team, plays a pivotal role. Of course, they are needed to convey new plans and guidance from Team One to the broader staff, but communication flows the other way as well – their proximity to day-to-day operations allows them to bring valuable insights and updates to Team One.

In the early stages of this approach, especially during the challenges posed by the rapid changes brought on by COVID-19, we discovered the importance of strategic communication. Recognizing that over-communication can be as detrimental as under-communication, we refined our approach. We streamlined information to smaller, digestible portions tailored to specific teams – be it the kennel team, tech team, surgery team, front staff, or doctors.

Communication Must Be Constant

In a veterinary practice, communication is an ongoing commitment that should evolve and change alongside your practice's needs, goals, and business structure.[7] Having communications systems in place is not enough. To truly understand the pulse of your practice, you have to go beyond surface-level inquiries. Instead of asking a generic "How's it going?" delve into specific areas, seeking feedback on recent changes or improvements. Ask open-ended questions like: "What did you think of the new surgery drop-off plan? How could we improve this?" If you just ask, "How's it going?" you will mostly just get the answer, "It's going okay," – and nothing gets improved. People need open-ended questions to think about what you're asking, and it helps them to dive further into an answer for you. In addition, you need to make sure they know their opinion matters and get feedback about the final decisions and how their input was taken into account in the plan.

Maintaining effective communication and collaboration is an iterative process. Complacency can lead to stagnation, so it's important that you commit to consistently poking and prodding at your systems. It's not about having a system that works and resting on your laurels; it's an ongoing dedication to refining and adapting your approach. I tell everyone that, in order to live up to our mission, we will always be evaluating our care and our systems. We will change them when needed, but at a thoughtful pace. It's equally important to know what and when the team can manage. If you push too much change at once, it will fail. This is where having more input is so helpful. The team will let you know if too much change is occurring and they cannot keep up. It's important to be able to say "no" to new changes sometimes if the timing isn't right.

Knowing what can be changed, and how much it can be changed, in a given time period comes with experience and depends on the skill level and commitment of the team. Every practice is different.

Sustaining Alignment Through Documentation

When working to maintain team unity, documentation[4] is a huge factor. At The Drake Center, we've cultivated an arsenal of tools. At the forefront is a document we call the "Drake Difference," which spells out exactly how we operate our hospital differently from the average practice. Conceived over two decades ago, this document has evolved into a dynamic, living expression of our values and commitments. We use documents like this as guideposts for how to be true to our mission. In addition, it makes a great training tool for new hires.

The Drake Center for Veterinary Care "Difference"

The Drake Center Mission is to provide the best medicine and surgery in a compassionate environment for our patients, and unsurpassed customer service for our clients. Everything we do is in support of this mission statement.

Unsurpassed Customer Service

We always treat you with kindness and respect. We listen to and address our client's concerns. We will always see your pet when it needs to be seen. We have extended hours, we are open seven days a week, drop-off appointments are available every day, and we will always follow up with you to make sure your pet is doing well. Our front office is composed of many long-term employees who will make sure you get the information and care you need. We continually update our service model to provide effective and efficient service and care.

Exceptional Standards of Care

The Drake Center is AAHA-accredited, which signifies we have met stringent quality standards in facilities and levels of care. Only 15% of all veterinary hospitals in the US meet this level of care. Our promise is to care for every patient as if they were our own pets. Our doctor and nursing staff-to-patient ratio is extremely high, and your pet receives individualized attention the entire time they are in our care. We are committed to optimal pain management and stress reduction during the visits, and in all recommendations. Our wellness care is customized to fit your pet and your family's best interests and welfare. There is no "one size fits all."

Highly Trained Medical Team

Many of our staff have been here for 10+ years. This translates into a highly experienced team of veterinary doctors and nursing staff. All new staff members go through a lengthy training process before they begin working with clients and caring for our patients. Our teams meet monthly, and our doctors have an additional monthly meeting to continue to share best practices and the most updated options for care. Every member of our team learns together and works together to better service our patients and their families. Our team approach means your pet's care will be exemplary.

Commitment to Client Education
Client education is a priority. We partner with you to understand your pet's needs and help formulate the best health care plan for your dog or cat. It is our expectation that you will not leave our hospital until you fully understand your pet's needs. In addition to our doctors' and technicians' discussions with you, we offer oral and written discharge instructions; an excellent library of hand-outs for your pet's specific needs; educational notebooks for our clients with puppies, kittens, and senior pets; and a website with a massive amount of supporting care information.

We Are Proud of Our Facility
A great deal of care goes into providing a veterinary care facility that is clean and odor-free. We strive to maintain our facility and are constantly improving our hospital to better serve our clients.

This statement of our differentiation is a powerful tool for recruitment and training of DVMs and staff, as well as attracting high-quality clientele who are well aligned with our mission. I encourage you to craft something similar for your practice that reflects your mission and values.

The Drake Difference isn't a static relic; it's a living, breathing entity that reflects the pulse of our practice. This document has weathered numerous adjustments and adaptations. In fact, just yesterday, I revisited it, inviting insights from eight individuals within my leadership team and beyond.

By seeking input from multiple perspectives, we ensure that the Drake Difference is not merely a top-down decree, but a shared expression of our collective values. The comments and suggestions we received provide a variety of insights, allowing us to fine-tune our guiding principles.

Documentation, including the Drake Difference, serves as a North Star for our team. In the constant ebb and flow of a veterinary practice, with new faces and changing dynamics, having a well-defined set of guiding principles becomes paramount. It's not just a manual; it's a compass that keeps us heading in the right direction.

The need for adaptation is a recurring theme in our approach. With a team that has seen growth, transitions, and evolving needs, we understand the importance of keeping our documentation fresh. The Drake Difference, like a well-tended garden, undergoes periodic pruning and nourishment, ensuring that it remains relevant and resonant.

Onboarding Excellence: Nurturing New Team Members

Onboarding new team members begins with hiring people who fit our culture. Chris, our manager, is extremely capable of finding culture fits for our practice. Her listening skills are extremely important in finding good fits for our practice. If you are interested only in skills, you will miss hiring people who will elevate your practice, and you may even wind up with some who detract.

Welcoming new team members into your established structure is a critical aspect of maintaining alignment. The key lies in embracing training as an integral part of your business culture. Recognize that technology evolves, processes are refined, and the best practices will shift over time. Therefore, training materials should not be static relics, but dynamic resources, constantly updated to reflect the latest insights and methodologies.

I believe that training staff is one of the most difficult aspects of owning a small business. You must hire well *and* train well to have a strong business. This is not easy, but it is doable with constant attention – even if done only in baby steps.

From traditional methods like mentoring and shadowing to modern tools such as videos and interactive programs, there are multiple ways to ensure that each newcomer is seamlessly integrated into the fabric of your aligned team. Promoting staff development and taking the time to teach and train newcomers can not only strengthen your team's capabilities while giving them greater autonomy in their roles, but also relieve some pressure off of doctors when new skills are learned and tasks can be delegated.[8]

Take the time to work out how you can improve your mentorship program in your hospital. It will pay off hugely over the long run. In addition, make sure you are utilizing all the benefits of today's technology for training. Many tasks that team members need to be taught can be learned via video. You can easily shoot training videos on an iPhone with no fuss. It's not about making the video look perfect; it's about delivering quality information. Utilizing videos allows new team members to get part of their training more passively. No one can train (or be trained) 8–10 hours a day. Utilizing written and video materials, along with mentoring and shadowing, allows a more palatable form of training for both the trainer and the trainee.

Navigating Accountability: Balancing Teamwork and Individual Responsibilities

Well-defined roles maintain a harmonious work environment. Each team member has specific responsibilities, ensuring that the collective effort aligns seamlessly with our overarching goals.

For instance, when our technicians prepare exam rooms, we have a methodical process for collecting history, addressing preventive care, and initiating necessary discussions before the doctor steps in. If any aspect is overlooked, accountability kicks in – not in anger, but in a constructive dialogue aimed at understanding and improvement. We ask our doctors to participate in training because they are working daily with many team members, and they are acutely aware of the team's skill levels. We utilize our DVMs' input to help with staff promotion and development. It can be as simple as emailing a few names of new staff to our DVMs and asking for their input on what areas they find are strong in these employees and what areas they may need more training. This very simple tool is so helpful for staff development and accountability.

Direct Confrontation with a Purpose

Maintaining accountability on a team is not about assigning blame, but rather understanding and correcting deviations from established protocols. If a surgery team member fails to complete assigned tasks, direct communication is key. The emphasis should be on a respectful inquiry: "Why wasn't this done, and what challenges did you face?" This approach fosters a culture where problems are addressed constructively, encouraging transparency and learning.

Confrontation, in this context, is not a negative term but a proactive way of addressing issues. Whether it's tardiness or incomplete tasks, a gentle but firm approach is crucial. For instance, if a team member is late, instead of expressing anger, ask them why they are late and engage in a dialogue about the importance of punctuality as well as some potential solutions. Make sure this team member understands the impact that their tardiness has on other members of the team. This proactive confrontation ensures that expectations are clear and deviations can be addressed promptly. It also lets the team members know what we expect in a respectful manner.

It's important to recognize that team members may have valid reasons for their actions, even if they deviate from the standard protocol. It's essential to listen and adjust policies accordingly when necessary. If a team member, burdened with multiple tasks, is unable to fulfill all responsibilities, this may be a time to reassess the distribution of workload in the hospital. This adaptability ensures that accountability is a two-way street. If you are hiring well, then it's safe to assume that your team members *want* to do the right thing and just need help figuring out how exactly to accomplish that.

The Client Experience: Efficient Team Coordination

A commitment to accountability should extend to optimizing the client experience. In a multi-doctor practice, clients may not always see the same veterinarian. At The Drake Center, we're open seven days a week, but our doctors work three to four days a week. Because our doctors have a system and we share practice guidelines, our clients quite often cannot distinguish between us! Clients may always request a specific doctor if they want to, but quite often, they prefer to be seen ASAP.

Efficiency is paramount, and it's important to focus on minimizing wait times. This is a consistent area of complaint that I see about other practices. Today's consumers are in a hurry for everything, and they often don't understand why things take time. This doesn't mean we should cut corners on care, but it does mean we should find ways to deliver great care efficiently.

Clients on-site and those on the phone should always be prioritized, showing them you are focused on their needs. Utilizing technology can be very helpful in alleviating wait times and creating efficiency. However, I am a very firm believer that human interaction is always the preferred method and the best way to establish a community of care and trust with clients. I have always said that

I will be in the ground before we utilize something cold and impersonal like a "phone tree" or automated phone system.

However, we do now utilize an online appointment scheduler for clients who prefer this method of setting appointments, and it is a wonderful system. It also allows phone receptionists to have more time for necessary conversations.

I recently was at a virtual AVMA Economic Summit, and one practice was so proud of its check-in and check-out process that was all done via a screen in the lobby. No humans are necessary. I will be in the ground before we allow someone to visit our practice without a personal welcome and goodbye.

Teamwork and Leadership

The essence of motivation in a veterinary practice should come from dedication to exceptional patient care. Observing the leadership team's relentless pursuit of excellence can serve as an inspiration for the entire team. It's about more than just completing daily tasks; it's about the sacrifices made to uphold the highest care standards. When this level of commitment is evident, it becomes a motivation for everyone in the practice.

Each team member's wholehearted contribution is essential. If a few team members are slacking off in a way that impacts your ability to deliver on your mission, it's crucial to address this promptly. The expectation should be for everyone to contribute their best; this promotes unity and shared responsibility.

Your leadership team should actively communicate and exemplify the practice's core values. When new members join, they should feel immersed in an environment where striving for excellence is the norm. The ambition to be part of a practice known for outstanding care can powerfully sustain motivation.

The influence of your leadership team's dedication and hard work extends throughout the practice. By championing these values, they create a domino effect, inspiring each team member to give their best. This creates a collective drive toward excellence.

Teamwork Is a Boon for Practice Owners and Pet Owners

Embracing the lesson of teamwork not only transforms the internal dynamics of a veterinary practice, but also yields significant benefits for practice owners[9] and, ultimately, pet owners.

Shared Accountability Eases the Burden

Teamwork redistributes the weight of responsibilities, ensuring that no single individual bears the brunt of challenges. Whether it's handling a difficult case or managing a negative review, the collective effort of the team lessens the stress on practice owners. Shared accountability becomes a powerful tool for navigating the complexities of the veterinary landscape.

Collective Problem Solving Delivers Better Outcomes

When faced with tough decisions or challenging situations, relying on a team of diverse perspectives enhances problem solving. Practice owners can tap into the collective wisdom of their teams to navigate intricate scenarios. The result is not just a resolution but an outcome shaped by collaboration, fostering a sense of achievement and shared success.

Elevated Quality of Patient Care

For pet owners, the benefits extend to elevated standards of care. In a collaborative environment where teamwork is ingrained in the practice culture, there's a shared commitment to providing exceptional service. This translates into improved patient care, reduced burnout among veterinary professionals, and an overall healthier working environment.

Mitigating Burnout: A Win for Pet Owners

A more collaborative practice also positively impacts pet owners and pets by mitigating burnout among veterinary professionals. When the workload and challenges are shared collectively, there's a positive ripple effect on the overall well-being of the veterinary team. This, in turn, leads to a more sustainable and fulfilling profession, ultimately benefiting the pets under their care.

Teamwork isn't just a professional strategy – it's a transformative approach that enriches the lives of practice owners, their teams, and, most importantly, the cherished pets who depend on our care. By fostering a culture of collaboration, the veterinary industry can embark on a journey toward resilience, improved well-being, and a shared commitment to excellence.

Build Your VPOS: Action Items for Teamwork

Evaluate Team Qualifications
Conduct an individual assessment of each team member's alignment with the practice's mission and core values.

- **Questions to Ponder:**
  - Do team members embody the positive qualities essential for a collaborative environment?
  - How well do the team's actions align with the practice's mission and commitment to patient care?
  - Is messaging and protocol consistent across the hospital, or are some team members "out of the loop"?
  - Is there any conflict between teams, such as "the front vs. the back"?

- **Action Steps:**
  - Identify which areas have strong alignment and which areas require improvement.
  - Develop a simple plan to reinforce teamwork through ongoing training and communication.
  - Make sure that you take at least one step forward on this plan at each of your staff meetings.

Invest in Team Study and Training

Choose two or three great books – I've recommended a few throughout this book, but you may have your own as well.

- Develop a reading plan for selected books with defined timelines.
- Facilitate interactive discussions during staff meetings to apply book concepts to real practice scenarios.

Implement Continuous Improvement

Reflect on the current culture of continuous improvement within the team.

- **Questions to Ponder:**
  - How often are progress and outcomes reviewed for continuous enhancement?
  - Is there an open feedback loop that encourages team members to suggest improvements?
  - When team members do suggest improvements, are they acted on promptly when possible, and are team members kept informed about any progress on addressing issues they have raised?
- **Action Steps:**
  - Reinforce the importance of providing constructive feedback during meetings.

- Ensure there is an easy way for team members to provide feedback and suggestions. This can be done through team surveys, one-on-one meetings, or a simple email. Keep in mind that some of your smartest employees may be introverts who are not comfortable making suggestions in front of a big group.
- Create a structured process for regular reviews with each team member, where their manager can go over what's working well, and what needs improvement.

References

1. Ji, H. and Yan, J. How team structure can enhance performance: team longevity's moderating effect and team coordination's mediating effect. Frontiers in Psychology [Internet]. 2020;11(1). https://doi.org/10.3389/fpsyg.2020.01873/full.
2. Lencioni, P. The Five Dysfunctions of a Team. San Francisco, CA: Pfeiffer; 2002.
3. Grove, A. High Output Management. Vintage; 1985.
4. Weinstein, P. Creating processes for a consistent, repeatable client experience [Internet]. DVM. 2018;360. Available from: https://www.dvm360.com/view/creating-processes-for-a-consistent-repeatable-client-experience
5. University of Maryland, Baltimore. Marketing Rule of Seven [Internet]. University of Maryland, Baltimore. Available from: https://www.umaryland.edu/cpa/rule-of-seven/
6. Covey, S. First Things First. Simon & Schuster; 2017.
7. Drake, M. Getting on the same page: proven communication strategies to align your team [Internet]. DVM. 2022;360. Available from: https://www.dvm360.com/view/getting-on-the-same-page-proven-communication-strategies-to-align-your-team

8. Surveyer, S. More than just a doctor: working with your team. The Canadian Veterinary Journal [Internet]. 2020;61(2):187–8. Available from: https://www.ncbi.nlm.nih.gov/pmc/articles/PMC6973215/

9. Drake, M. Why team building makes all the difference in your practice and how to do it right [Internet]. DVM. 2022;360. Available from: https://www.dvm360.com/view/why-team-building-makes-all-the-difference-in-your-practice-and-how-to-do-it-right

8

Agility

> Stay flexible.
> Always have a plan – but never be afraid to adapt your plan to new situations.

One week before the financial market meltdown of 2008, I had paid a down payment on a cabin in Mammoth Mountain. I remember this so clearly because I was truly scared about what to do. I still bought the cabin, but I decided to focus all my attention on my practice to ensure it weathered the storm successfully.

Any crisis is a great time to reassess how we do business. It was a very scary time, as anyone who owned a practice at that time could attest. But even more unsettling than the financial meltdown was the release of the first iPhone. Because I read the WSJ daily, I was keenly aware of how

---

Veterinary Leadership: A Practical Guide for Practice Owners and Managers,
First Edition. Michele Drake.
© 2025 John Wiley & Sons, Inc. Published 2025 by John Wiley & Sons, Inc.

little I knew about technology, but it was clear that the iPhone was going to change the world as we knew it.

Agility is the ability to think and move quickly. I immediately started reading about how the iPhone was going to change our customers' behavior. Our clients now had 24/7 access to information, but I still wanted to be the one to bring it to them. That way they would retain their trust in my practice, rather than relying on questionable online sources. This was the beginning of my foray into digital marketing, which has become a key part of the success of The Drake Center in the years since 2008.

Agile Leadership Is Vital in Unprecedented Times

While I know it's just one of many challenges we've all faced in this industry, it's impossible to start this chapter with anything but the COVID-19 pandemic. To say it was a time of uncertainty in our industry is the understatement of the year.

My practice is in California and while this is not intended to be a political book, let's just say we have a unique government in this state that no one would call "business-friendly." I'm sure many practice owners in California and other states faced similar issues with constant changes in regulations from both the government and our certifying organizations.

From pivoting to curbside service to "bubble staffing" to constantly needing to re-plan the schedule when people were either ill or caring for family members who were ill, this period was a real challenge.

Flexibility was the critical factor that allowed The Drake Center to pivot quickly and efficiently. It wasn't about being reactive, but about being aware and having systems in place that allowed us to make continual adjustments. It required us to have a team that was used to participating in decisions and a communication system that allowed for optimal sharing of updated information. Another factor that really helped us during this time was to always manage from a central philosophy that we work on the things we can control, and we remain aware of the others while acknowledging what we can't control. Frustration and hand-wringing are useless. Accept what you cannot change, and work on the things you can change. There are always plenty of positive responses in any situation.

Among many other innovations, we:

- Created a remote phone support team – I had a couple of older employees who simply couldn't safely be in the practice, but they were happy to keep working from home to take care of our increasing volume of calls.
- Installed a Ring camera system in the parking lot so the receptionist could visualize the flow of client traffic and react quickly by bringing out meds or food, or helping facilitate the next appointment.
- We had only 10 parking places, which was nowhere near enough for our traffic flow. To solve this, we gave out Starbucks coupons to our clients so they could wait there across the street, allowing us to keep the traffic moving in and out quickly.
- Used Facetime to communicate with clients in their cars about their pet's exam and our plan.
- Launched a text-based client management app. We found a tool from the hospitality industry that allowed us to create automated text conversations with our curbside clients, helping reduce our insane phone call volume by more than 50% while speeding up service for our clients.
- Pivoted to Zoom-based team meetings to ensure that all team members could be kept in the loop of new developments even when not in the practice.

As a result of these efforts, while many practices booked out two or more months for new patients or even just simply shut their doors, The Drake Center thrived. It was a crazy time, but I'm proud to say we grew substantially during the pandemic, including hiring four additional doctors and 20 additional staff, and even opening a second annex location to handle all the new patients. Having a system in place that "works *on* the practice" and a great flow of communication allows us to respond to any challenge. COVID-19 was just like any other challenge we've dealt with in our history – just bigger and longer in duration.

In addition to leaning on our systems and communication, I also kept aware of the economy, consumer behavior, and external influences. For me, this meant keeping a daily eye on the *WSJ*, AVMA, AAHA, and other veterinary and business news outlets. Staying aware empowers us to make strategic decisions and navigate the storm with resilience and creativity.

While, of course, we're all hoping there isn't another pandemic anytime soon, I believe that having these systems in place allows a kind of flexibility that is vital for navigating many other types of challenges that we will all inevitably face in the future. Managing the practice during a very volatile time was challenging but not impossible.

Embracing Evolution: Overcoming Resistance to Change

In life, change is the only constant. Yet DVMs are often very resistant to it. I've witnessed many instances where this resistance proved detrimental to practices' well-being and success.

Let's start with the struggle to find "adequately trained staff." Finding skilled professionals, including RVTs, assistants, and receptionists, had always been a challenge, even before the pandemic hit. The shortage wasn't a new phenomenon; it just got a lot worse.[1] Finding a qualified RVT was extremely tough before COVID-19; it was impossible during COVID-19.

When talking with fellow veterinarians during this time, I urged them to shift their perspective. The traditional approach to recruitment and retention needed a refresh.

Many practice owners I spoke with simply beat their heads against the wall, complaining that there were no good people available and continuing to struggle with too few staff – but they were unwilling to change their approach in the face of changing reality.[2]

The reality was, with the traffic to veterinary clinics in the United States increasing by 4.5% from 2019 to 2020, and then again by 6.5% between January and June of 2021,[3] there was just no way there would be enough trained people anytime soon to take care of all those pets. We were going to have to approach this differently.

So we did our best with the circumstances and adjusted continually. We adopted a proactive strategy with two main components:

1. Accept that not every employee is a "lifer" – and plan your training accordingly.
2. Hire for culture fit, train for skills, and create new roles where needed.

Accept That Not Every Employee Is a "Lifer" – And Plan Your Training Accordingly

When I started my career, the expectation was to hire a set number of employees who would stay with the practice for many years – possibly the entirety of their careers. This has completely changed today. The veterinary workforce has evolved, with a significant influx of individuals in their twenties, many of whom are just "checking out" the field and maybe planning for veterinary or tech school later. At The Drake Center, we have the added challenge of San Diego now being considered the most unaffordable city in the United States. So we have issues with our younger employees being able to afford to live here over the long term.

We recognized that the tenure of these young professionals might be relatively short, but their value was undeniable – and they were essential during the staffing shortage created by COVID-19.

Instead of bemoaning their transient nature, we embraced it. We tailored our training programs to rapidly equip them with skills they could use *now* in order to contribute meaningfully – without spending six months training someone who might only be with us for two years. We took a pragmatic approach: how we feel about this trend is frankly irrelevant; it's a reality, and the sooner we find a way to work with it, the better we will do as a practice.

I should mention that this applies to a specific subset of staff. My practice manager has been with me for over 30 years, and we have near-zero attrition of DVMs. We have several RVTs and receptionists who have been with the practice for over 20 years. So, of course, we want to invest as much time and energy as possible in retaining these higher-skilled team members that our practices depend on. But at the same time, we need to be okay with some turnover at the lower levels, and we need a system to minimize the impact of that turnover.

Hire for Culture Fit, Train for Skills, and Create New Roles Where Needed

Recognizing that there simply were not enough already-skilled people available, we adjusted our expectations and pivoted toward hiring for culture fit and training for skills. The good news is that while there may be a shortage of RVTs, there are millions of young people who are smart, kind, responsible pet lovers. Many of them would probably fit in well at your practice. Once we accepted this new approach, we found there were plenty of candidates to consider for every opening we had.

Of course, we aimed for A+ culture fit in every hire, but with everything going on at the time, we had to make some compromises. Some hires were a bit short on communication skills or missing some specific knowledge we would normally look for. But, we remained committed to meeting our hiring goals to support our community, and this meant we got very creative with training to fill any gaps.

We also created new roles that weren't "traditional" positions; rather, they were tailored to support various departments that were stretched thin. Some became integral supporting members of our surgery team, while others helped along the front line, ensuring smooth operations in critical areas. The point is to "think outside the box." Just because we have had very specific roles for years does not mean that we cannot adjust and change the roles to fit our needs.

- We created the role of "surgery team assistant" (STA), who helped with restraint, patient movement, and other low-skilled jobs to support the surgery team.
- We created a "treatment room assistant" (TRA) who simply helped the exam room team with restraint and setting up lab tests and samples, assisting clients in and out of the building.
- We also created a "receptionist assistant" who aided in running back and forth from the parking lot and handling some calls to communicate with clients.

We were specific with the job descriptions based on what the team needed. We created the new job descriptions, trained people for them quickly, and put them to work to support the team.

These roles didn't demand a very high level of skill, but they did require individuals who resonated with our culture. Creating more low-skill positions to support the higher-skilled employees helped us deal with increased volume while avoiding burnout. Many hospitals have "tiers" for their employees, which seems like a great method for training and managing pay scales as well.

Of course, these two strategies are intimately connected. By creating more lower-skill roles, we accommodate a more transient labor force without incurring huge costs from turnover. In addition, the team is on board with training because they know these new team members will support them in valuable ways when they are performing their higher-skill jobs. In addition, this empowers the more skilled employees to share their knowledge and become stronger team members in the process. Training someone else is a great way to solidify your own skills and reassess the job at the same time. If the new employees engage and perform well, we begin to move them up the skills ladder according to their abilities.

Rising to the Occasion in Alignment with Our Mission

By being agile in our hiring and adjusting our approach to align with the immediate demands of local pet owners, we were able to rise to the occasion and keep up with the increased demand.

At the time, I honestly wasn't trying to do anything heroic. I was just focused on delivering on our mission and continuing to be there for our community.

As I've shared this story with other practice owners, though, I've realized that our approach was actually quite unusual. In times of stress, take a breath, gather your team around you, take the time to problem solve, and then act. Everyone faced challenges during this time, but many failed to adapt sufficiently or chose to take a less-active approach. The only true failure is not taking the time to be objective, assess the situation, and make a plan. Take the time to work on your practice, not just in your practice.

A major corporate practice right down the street from The Drake Center simply closed down completely because it could not be flexible enough to find solutions and stay open. Or possibly their staff felt no loyalty toward them? Similar things happened in many other practices in San Diego to one degree or another, such as practices closing on random days, reducing hours, or booking out eight or more weeks for appointments. I've even seen some practices putting big notices on their websites saying, "Sorry, we are not accepting new patients."

All of this led more and more pet owners in our community to come to The Drake Center, where our mantra was "fit in patients who need to be seen – we need to support our community." This led to unprecedented growth. If you're wondering whether the staff got tired, the answer is "Yes, sometimes." However, we reacted quickly to these needs by hiring and adding shifts, and I began to build out more space for us, as well.

The annex we added to our building in an adjacent commercial space, added six more exam rooms and allowed us to increase the number of patients we were able to accommodate on our schedule each day. This new space was nicknamed "the spa." Because of its open design and beauty, it became a favored working space for the team. We grew and invested in our team and our space and updated many ways of doing business. The increase in the size of our team allows for more services and opportunities for our team. The additional four doctors we added brought more diversity of knowledge and more flexibility to our schedule for all doctors. We've always had the DVM culture of working hard, but everyone also gets to take off whatever time they need. I have never denied a vacation request if the dates are not flexible, such as for a family reunion or special trip. In addition, we continue to update everyone's schedule requests as their lives change, such as a new baby or when kids go back to school. We do our best to accommodate everyone. We always figure it out, and we always work together to cover shifts.

So much of the world was closed during COVID-19; there was not a lot to do except worry, so we chose to be a mission-driven business and take care of our patients. In addition, we did take extra care of our staff. We did not ask people to work overtime, we brought in meals more often, and we gave cash bonuses to acknowledge the very hard work and diligence the team provided while they were working. By focusing on our mission, The Drake Center offered a respite from the insanity of COVID-19 for our team.

Resisting Change Can Hurt Your Practice

Clinging to outdated perspectives can have profound consequences. I recently engaged with a group that exemplified a rigid, inflexible mindset, and their story serves as a cautionary tale for practices reluctant to embrace change.

During the challenging days of COVID-19, many veterinary hospitals chose a path that left me bewildered: in spite of unprecedented demand for our services, they opted to *downsize*. This seemed senseless. Phones were ringing incessantly with pet owners in desperate need – the very reason we all entered this profession. While I don't advocate for burning out your team, as it turned out, our team *didn't* burn out – we adapted, worked diligently, and persevered through the increase in volume.

To be honest, the fourth tenet of our culture, "fun," was hard to keep alive during these very busy times. We had to remind ourselves of the importance of keeping this going even during very tough times. On the other hand, our practice was inundated with a massive influx of puppies. If you can't find joy and fun with puppies coming into your practice every day, it might be time to rethink your career choices.

For those who resist change, running a successful and thriving veterinary practice becomes an uphill battle. The ability to adapt when necessary is not just a survival skill; it's the essence of sustainability and growth in our profession. As we navigate a dynamic industry and consumer environment, the choice becomes clear: evolve or risk becoming irrelevant, overshadowed by practices that embrace change and thrive in the face of adversity.

Navigating Change: Remember the Seven-Times Rule

Recently, we initiated a change involving our second tech's role (the second in for the day) in overseeing boarding patients. We have a kennel team, but many of them are younger and less experienced, so we want a tech to check in with the kennel team and have eyes on every boarding patient twice a day. It's a subtle change, but a crucial one in ensuring the well-being of our patients.

The second tech verifies records, ensures updates are accurate and, most importantly, offers support to our kennel team. This keeps the team more connected and helps prevent "silos" where individuals or small parts of the team have key information that is not being shared with others. We've learned to ask specific questions, recognizing the need to go beyond a generic offer of "How can I help?"

When we make subtle but specific changes to how we operate daily (always based upon our mission statement), it still requires significant follow-up to ensure the new changes are fully in place and being acted upon. This doesn't mean we don't trust our staff to get it right; it's simply knowing that these types of changes require several follow-ups (often seven or more) to make sure they are being done, as we all agreed was best for patient care. It's important not to get frustrated, but just to realize that it takes a while to get a new routine to become the norm.

You'll have changes to make in your practice as you grow. Agility is vital to your success, but it can create confusion. Follow the seven times rule – don't get frustrated if your team doesn't "get it" immediately when you make a change. Persist in communicating about the new process, and they'll catch up in time.

Agility Includes Listening to Your Team

Many practice owners – including myself – are "drivers" and have strong personalities. We may seem hard to push back against. However, in fact, I absolutely love it when someone tells us something isn't working and they have a suggestion. When your team comes up with ideas, it means they care and are thinking about your processes as well. This is awesome! I love to be challenged to make things better for patients, clients, and staff.

While I drive the overarching vision for the practice, I acknowledge my limitations in certain areas. For instance, when discussing topics like using technology, I lean on the expertise of my team, especially our manager, Chris. She is much more attuned to the uses and needs of technology, so she leads those discussions.

In those moments, my role shifts from the primary innovator to a facilitator, ensuring that the momentum isn't lost. I guide the team through action steps, emphasizing the importance of not letting good ideas languish. It's this collaborative spirit that defines our culture of innovation – a dynamic interplay of leadership-driven vision and collective problem-solving prowess.

Response, Not Reaction: Avoid Reactivity in Your Practice

We will always have situations in our practices that we need to respond to and handle. While it's vital to be agile and adjust when it's needed, not every situation requires a change in policy or process.

The key is to distinguish between a knee-jerk reaction and a thoughtful, strategic response. It's tempting to react to a mistake that was made or a client that got angry with our team. However, it's best to put a little thought and even some reconnaissance into the issue before making a decision.

When faced with an upset client or a mistake, resist the urge to immediately make a policy change; first, focus on collecting information. The goal is not to assign blame, but to gather enough information to determine whether a mistake was made or if a policy adjustment is necessary. The following approach sets the stage for creating sustainable solutions that prevent similar issues in the future.

1. **Approach the Staff Member(s) Involved:** Collect information and calmly discuss the situation, understanding the steps taken and the individuals involved. It takes time, but this deliberate

approach is essential to understand the context and make informed decisions.

2. **Determine If a Change Really Needs to Be Made:** Quite often, nothing actually needs to be done – and if you had immediately taken action based on your first "gut reaction," you might have ended up creating a problem where there really wasn't one. If you determine that action is truly needed, only then go ahead.

3. **Rectify the Situation:** If an apology is necessary, it's offered sincerely. If confrontation is required, it is done constructively and with the intention of fostering growth. The key is to address the issue head-on, deal with it effectively, and then move forward. Conflict-aversion is a widespread problem in our field. I've often heard DVMs say they are "too nice to confront that person about that issue." In reality, avoiding confrontation is not "nice," as it often results in burdening the entire team with continuing dysfunction.

4. **Adjust Your Plans Going Forward Through Policy and Communication:** When you do find that action is needed, share that information at your next leadership meeting and/or general staff meeting.

Informed Decision-Making Through Continuous Learning

Staying ahead of trends and changes in the veterinary field is vital for informed decision-making. I recommend digital formats such as *Today's Veterinarian*, AVMA, and *DVM360*. These sources not only cover industry trends, but also provide valuable insights and articles. By staying informed, you can anticipate trends, identify potential challenges, and adjust your approach proactively.

I particularly appreciate the current AVMA president, Dr. Rena Carlson, and her focus on the problem of reactivity in veterinary medicine. We need to respond to the shortage of DVMs and other industry challenges with a strategic, thoughtful response rather than succumbing to reactivity and panic. By continuously learning and engaging with industry trends, you can ensure your practice remains resilient and responsive to the evolving needs of your community.

Trends and Technology in Veterinary Medicine

While most people in the industry are talking about a shortage of DVMs, at this exact moment, there are ten new veterinary schools in construction, and others are expanding. Industry-driven changes, such as reduced requirements for the veterinary–patient relationship in medication distribution, further complicate this paradox. A strategic approach involves examining the data at hand and anticipating the consequences of this massive expansion. In the next 5–10 years, there's a real possibility of an oversupply of veterinarians, leading to a shift in dynamics and priorities within the profession. While many are currently panicking about a shortage of veterinary professionals, they may soon be panicking because there are too many!

The influx of veterinarians is not just a numerical concern; it reflects a broader shift in the profession's values. While financial considerations have become prominent, there's an acknowledgment that this trend is unsustainable. The focus on money is expected to evolve, paving the way for a reevaluation of priorities and a return to the core mission of serving animals and their owners.

The industry's trajectory is shaped by diverse stakeholders with varying interests. The push for reduced regulations by entities like Walmart reflects a commercial interest, leveraging the current climate for profit. A thoughtful analysis of these dynamics is essential to navigate the complexities and ensure that decisions align with the best interests of veterinarians, their patients, and the profession as a whole.

Embracing Technology with Caution

In discussing technology, it's imperative to address the fine line between innovation and exploitation. While technology has the potential to enhance agility and efficiency, we also need to be mindful of platforms that capitalize on our vulnerabilities. When we get stressed, we want solutions, and we do not always follow and trust our instincts as much as we should. We often assume that the industry may know more than we do. Because we are siloed in our practices, we have to have great resources to turn to and great systems in place to make sound decisions.

It's essential to dissect the broader question: *How can technology be harnessed responsibly to elevate veterinary medicine and make your practice more agile, innovative, and effective?* Our answer lies within striking the delicate balance between profit and purpose[4] in our technology use.

I believe that every practice is different in its needs and wants, so there is no "one-size-fits-all" solution. However, having a system for dealing with issues and opportunities before a stressful time allows us to make good decisions. I rely upon the AVMA and AAHA as places to begin. However, we must also remember that many of those in our governing bodies do not currently run a practice, and their motivations may be different when developing recommendations. Nonetheless, we generally get good input from them. I also greatly lean upon my CPA and members of my VMG group when considering a new technology or major equipment. Getting information from a wide swath of people and groups helps to make a well-rounded decision. Of course, I use the input of the team to make the final decision.

Discerning Practical Innovation from "Band-Aid" Solutions

The integration of technology into a veterinary practice can be a powerful tool when applied thoughtfully. The challenge lies in distinguishing between a helpful technological solution and a mere band-aid that may divert attention from fundamental issues in the practice. I believe that sometimes the industry may be recommending things to sell to us that provide an expensive band-aid but do not improve our delivery of care or service.

A very simple case in point is the "phone tree." When people call a business, their vast preference is to have a human answer and help them with their questions or needs. When phone trees became popular, I told my staff I would have to be dead before we used this in our practice. Rather than hire and train capable people to answer their phones and interact with patients, some owners chose these systems and have eliminated much of the human element associated with contacting their practice.

While there are many common issues that practice owners face, there are an equal number of voices in the industry telling you that they have a solution (for a price). I believe that we can find a better way to manage these issues in our practices without always looking for an outside solution that may be a quick fix ... again, assuming that you have a sound method for managing your practice and take the time to work *on* your practice.

At the same time, technology that enhances our client's experience and provides efficiency can be a blessing. For example, many clients prefer the option of online booking. It is becoming a standard in many professions. It's great when we can offer online booking for convenience, along with a human to answer the phone when needed.

Even though we felt online booking would be a great enhancement to our service, we didn't go into it blindly. We conducted sessions with the entire team, detailing the nuances of managing this new service. Breakout sessions allowed for tailored discussions, addressing specific concerns and questions. This collaborative approach ensured that every team member felt equipped to handle the change.

Our doctors were actively involved in the process. Their insights were sought at every stage, ensuring that the system adjustments didn't compromise the quality of patient care. Regular feedback loops were established to address any issues promptly and refine our approach based on practical experience.

The journey toward implementing online booking required more time and prep due to our business structure. However, keeping the key players of the front staff and the DVMs well informed and a part of our decision of how we would use this new system ensured it was rolled out successfully.

Aligning Technology with Actual Needs

To ensure that new technology serves as a genuine solution, it's essential to consult individuals with expertise in the field. In our case, a technology-savvy friend played a pivotal role in guiding us toward a text-based chatbot solution during COVID-19. We needed help to deal with the volume of calls required to manage curbside service, which was triple the volume we had before. We didn't adopt new tech for its own sake; we focused on addressing a real and immediate need within our practice.

The goal is not to react to perceived weaknesses (or "weaknesses" being pointed out by someone with a product to sell you) – but rather to proactively serve clients by aligning technology with their evolving needs.

The current buzz around telemedicine prompts a crucial question: *Does adopting this technology genuinely enhance patient and client service? Or is it driven by the desire of tech companies to gain market share in our industry?* There is just so much desire by industry and investors to "get a piece of the veterinary action." We need to be aware of the motives underlying this interest in our profession and what the results will be if we let these interests take over.

Telemedicine, while a valuable tool, needs to be monitored for its true benefits and the intentions of many dipping into this very lucrative area of technology. In addition to being sold to veterinarians as a tool, telemedicine is now also being sold to consumers as an option instead of a true VCPR. Of course, this is state-dependent, but many states, including California, are adjusting their VCPR definition in response to the high COVID-19 demands. However, these trends are already shifting again. My concern is for my profession. We use telemedicine as a tool at the Drake Center but not as any sort of replacement for our care. It is a tool, and that is all. None of us pretends to believe that it replaces the massive benefit of in-person patient care.

In the first iteration of the Veterinary Telemedicine guidelines published on the Canadian Veterinary Medical Association[5] (CVMA) website in April 2020, telemedicine was explicitly described as a complementary tool for veterinary medicine, not a replacement. Further updates to the guidelines only reinforced this notion.[6] We must use this as a reminder for all adoptions of technology within our field; we cannot let anything replace a true VCPR, and must instead focus on the tools and technologies that empower us to improve them.

In essence, the key is to approach technology with a discerning eye, avoiding reactionary adoption and instead aligning it with the authentic needs and expectations of clients and patients. This approach ensures that technology serves as a true asset, enhancing the efficiency and effectiveness of our veterinary practice.

Remote Reception – Pros and Cons

Another example of industry entering our profession is remote reception. While remote reception may be a temporary stop-gap, it may not be compatible with the practice's ethos over the long term. Similar to telemedicine, this is another technology that isn't inherently good or bad, but is very dependent on how it's deployed.

In my practice, we had some "retired" team members who came back to help us with remotely answering calls. They were already familiar with the practice's systems and culture. This was a great solution and did improve our efficiency.

There are also some practices that set up dedicated "phone rooms" with their own employees so that the front desk is handling only in-person clients and not bouncing back and forth to the phones or leaving people on hold. Again, this is often a good solution.

On the other hand, many businesses promote fully outsourcing the reception role to an off-site third party (often offshore), whose team members will not be fully familiar with how that practice runs. I don't recommend this approach. It's much better just to find and hire quality people and train them to do this job in your practice. Training is hard and time-consuming, but it's necessary for good patient care and client service.

This thoughtful approach to innovation applies to many areas of the practice, not just technology. Embracing an entrepreneurial mindset involves not only adapting to change but also proactively driving it. The agility to pivot, innovate, and modify business models will position your practice to navigate challenges effectively.

Mission-Driven Transformation: Aligning Change with Purpose

For practice owners hesitant about change, the key question is: *What's best for the practice?* The simple answer is to always align change with your practice's mission statement. If the practice's mission is to provide unsurpassed customer service, then embracing technological advancements that support this mission is worthwhile.

The ripple effect of agility and innovation extends beyond the practice owners to the entire industry. By staying attuned to advancements in patient care, such as digital radiology and dental rads, laparoscopic procedures, and so on, practices contribute to elevating the standard of veterinary care. Pet owners benefit directly from these advancements, receiving the best possible care for their beloved companions.

The journey toward agility and innovation is a holistic endeavor. It goes beyond adopting technology for its own sake; it's about cultivating a mindset that constantly seeks ways to enhance patient care, support clients, and uphold the mission that defines the practice's existence.

Build Your VPOS: Action Steps for Agility

Assess and Adapt
- **Reflection Questions:**
  - How adaptable is your practice to emerging trends and changing needs?
  - Do you have a defined process for considering new technologies or changes in your practice?
  - Do you feel "plugged in" to trends and new developments in veterinary medicine?
  - Are there changes in your practice, whether to personnel, processes, or plans, that you probably should have made, but have been putting off?
- **Action Steps:**
  - Make a habit of consistently reading the latest issues of high-quality publications in veterinary medicine, so you can keep your ear to the ground for new developments.
  - Assess your practice's use of technology. Are you taking advantage of new technologies that could help you deliver better care and service? Are there any technologies you've adopted that might not be serving your mission and should be changed?
  - Consider creating a "task force" in your practice to monitor industry trends and propose ways to adapt.

References

1. Petervary, N., Pritchard, C., Esparza-Trujillo, J. and Gopee, N. Veterinary Staffing Shortages and Potential Solutions During the COVID-19 Pandemic. Laboratory Animal Science Professional; 2020.
2. Drake, M. Navigating talent shortages [Internet]. DVM 360. 2023;54(7):50. Available from: https://www.dvm360.com/view/navigating-talent-shortages
3. Salois, M. and Golab, G. Are We in a Veterinary Workforce Crisis? [Internet]. American Veterinary Medical Association; 2021. Available from: https://www.avma.org/javma-news/2021-09-15/are-we-veterinary-workforce-crisis
4. Dunn, L. Striking a balance between profit and purpose. DVM 360 [Internet]. 2024;55(3):32–2. Available from: https://www.dvm360.com/view/striking-a-balance-between-profit-and-purpose
5. Chalhoub, S. Veterinary telemedicine [Internet]. Canadian Veterinary Medical Association; 2020 Available from: https://www.canadianveterinarians.net/media/ililtnnn/cvma-veterinary-telemedicine-guidelines.pdf
6. Kastelic, J. and Ogilvie, T. Veterinary telemedicine is not only here to stay, it's poised to grow and likely exponentially. The Canadian Veterinary Journal = La revue veterinaire canadienne 2021;62(12):1277–9.

9

Communications and Community

> Understand what "marketing" really means – and do it!

When COVID hit, I spent every day collecting information from WSJ, national news channels, CVMA, and AVMA. America and the world were in a crisis, and the information was panic-inducing for most people. I started to communicate with my team via emails, postings, and Zoom meetings. My team trusted me to distill the information and let them know how we were going to respond. Also, the door was open to discuss with us any fears or issues they may have personally. The calm in my practice during COVID and the amazing response of my team are reflections of the trust that had been built long ago, but it was that stream of communication that held us all together. It was an important reminder

---

Veterinary Leadership: A Practical Guide for Practice Owners and Managers, First Edition. Michele Drake.
© 2025 John Wiley & Sons, Inc. Published 2025 by John Wiley & Sons, Inc.

that you cannot over-communicate important pieces of information.
The important information includes where your practice is now, where it
is going, and how it is going to get there. Keep your team informed.

When your team is fully aligned, you can also communicate more
effectively with your community, and your local pet owners will want
to be part of your practice. My community quickly learned that The
Drake Center was here for them and their pets and that we were commit-
ted to delivering on our mission in spite of the challenges brought on by
COVID. This led us to unprecedented growth that has continued even
after the pandemic, as we built amazing goodwill by being there for our
community.

When I launched my practice back in 1992, I realized that creating a successful practice would require not only having a clear
mission and vision, but also making that mission known to people
in my community.

The conversation about marketing often elicits a collective
sigh among veterinarians, and it's understandable. We're passionate about animals, not necessarily digital strategies. Yet, the reality
is that marketing is an integral part of running a successful veterinary business, and its potential to connect us with our community
is immense.

I've found that many practice owners greatly misunderstand
what "marketing" really means. For many, when they think of marketing, they think of a used-car salesman on their TV shouting at
them about his "crazy low prices" or something. While that might
technically be called marketing, it's not what I'm talking about
here, and it's not what works for a veterinary practice.

What Is Marketing, Really?

To me, marketing could be best defined as: *Knowing who you are*
as a practice and making this known to your employees, clients, and
community.

When you really understand your own mission, vision, and brand, and when you communicate this authentically and effectively on every channel of interaction with the public, you will attract the right kind of clients that will help you build a successful practice.

The Evolution of Marketing Strategies

As I reflect on the evolution of our marketing program at The Drake Center, it's clear that staying current involves a continuous process of listening, learning, and embracing change. Our journey from the Yellow Pages to the digital space is a testament to the importance of staying ahead of the curve.

When I acquired my first practice in the early '90s, the landscape was different. Visibility was a challenge, and the Yellow Pages played a crucial role in establishing our presence. A well-crafted brochure, open houses, and community involvement were our primary strategies. Those were simpler times, but as technology advanced, so did the means of reaching our audience.

The turning point came in 2008, a year that marked significant economic and consumer behavior shifts. Recognizing the need for change, I sought the expertise of Harley Orion, a client and friend who owned a digital marketing agency (now the CEO of Genius-Vets). I asked him to come teach my team about this new reality of the digital world. He generously showed up every two weeks for a few months to spend about an hour with us, explaining the very basics of the new digital world and the impact of the iPhone. Our clients now had all the information from the internet at their fingertips any time any place. It was a paradigm shift, and I, admittedly, had very limited understanding at the time.

Armed with this new knowledge, we took the first steps into the digital world. A new website became our cornerstone, optimized for mobile devices as smartphones became ubiquitous. The process was gradual, a series of incremental advancements rather than a radical overhaul. Each step brought us closer to understanding how to connect with our audience in the digital sphere.

A Great Brand Attracts the Right Clients – And Helps You Avoid the Wrong Clients

Also, keep in mind that *a great brand both attracts and repels*. A great example is Harley-Davidson motorcycles. People are either Harley people or aren't, and they know it.

Another great example is Nordstrom – when you enter their store, you have certain expectations about the experience based on the brand they have created through their marketing communications. You expect great service, you expect high-quality products, and you expect to spend a decent amount of money there. You don't wander into a Nordstrom, thinking you're going into a Target or a Walmart. Those brands aren't bad, they're just different, and they are targeting different clients.

When I started The Drake Center, I had the vision of being "the Nordstrom of veterinary medicine." I wanted to create a place that inspired people. This meant crafting a narrative that was authentic to my vision and would resonate with both my team and the community we served.

The digital landscape was very different in 1992 than it is today. Yet the core principles remain unchanged – a clear vision, a passionate team, and a commitment to exceptional care. Back then, the goal was simple: Let people know what sets us apart, not just as a veterinary clinic but as a hub of compassionate, top-notch service.

Today, at The Drake Center, nestled in a mature community with a high density of veterinary practices, the landscape demands a different strategy. With 11 doctors and over 50 dedicated employees, our mission endures – delivering exceptional care. The challenge, however, lies in standing out amid the multitude of veterinary options in the area.

Digital marketing is the way we reach people who are not in our building, especially potential new clients. I have a vision in my head where, given the slow growth in my area, there are probably about 20 people a week who are seeking a new veterinarian within my service area. I want every single one of them to find their way to The Drake Center. This vision has heightened the importance of a robust digital presence, a strategic necessity if we want people to know who we are and what we do.

The Symbiosis of Marketing and Mission

I believe that marketing is part of running a disciplined business. And before you market well, you always have to go back to thinking about who you are and what you do that makes you different. Every time you think about your mission and values and how you communicate this to the community, you make yourself a stronger business.[1]

Your practice's digital presence should be the embodiment of your brand in the online space, reflecting who you are and what you stand for. It's the visual and informational gateway through which potential staff and clients form their first impressions. Aligning your digital presence with your mission is a necessity. It's very odd to me that so many practices with great cultures and great patient care have generic websites full of stock photos that don't say anything unique about the practice. This is a vital opportunity to engage with the community that is being missed.

One common misconception I've observed is the tendency to view a website merely as a digital brochure. The truth is that it should be a dynamic force driving your business forward. Digital marketing and social media play pivotal roles in staying relevant in today's world. When I speak at events or conferences, it's apparent that many veterinarians haven't fully grasped this concept. The discomfort in this space is palpable, and I get it. It's unfamiliar territory, and not everyone is comfortable navigating it.

To overcome this hurdle, I often emphasize the importance of connecting the dots between veterinarians and their clients. A website is not just a static page; it's a conduit for engagement. Search engine optimization (SEO) and compelling content can be the difference between a closed-door and a welcoming community. I've seen firsthand that bridging this gap can be a challenge, but it's a challenge worth undertaking. Then, there is the vital importance of having informational content on your website for your clients and potential clients. This is how we provide a service for our clients and the public by providing information they want for their pets. People will always be looking for pet health information online. Too often, instead of finding a local veterinarian, they end up on an e-commerce site or a random blog. Either we, as DVMs, must provide this information, or someone else with less-than-perfect motives will.

Creating an ecosystem of optimized information on a practice website and authentically showcasing a clinic's mission and values has driven results for hundreds of practices around the country,[2] displaying the need for embracing digital marketing tactics despite any discomfort or hesitations we may have due to unfamiliarity.

Internal Consistency: A Crucial Element of Trust

Envision this scenario: A potential client visits a practice's website and is captivated by the warm and friendly images of their team in action. They decide to pay a visit to the practice, only to encounter a different reality – crabby attitudes and a cluttered hospital. That incongruence can shatter expectations and erode trust.

For my practice, the website is a canvas where we paint an authentic picture of who we are. The images on the site are real snapshots of our daily activities, capturing the genuine essence of our practice. We are not projecting an idealized version – we are demonstrating how we are special. Like a website for a high-end restaurant or a stylish hotel, our site serves as a preview, preparing potential clients for the experience they can anticipate. Our website is more than a digital brochure – it's a window into our practice culture. We showcase not just our expertise but the warmth, cleanliness, and camaraderie that define us.

Our commitment to transparency extends beyond the virtual space. External marketing efforts, from community events to online campaigns, are rooted in our mission.

Weaving Community Threads

Community engagement has always been an important and consistent way we align our mission and culture with what we do outside the practice. I was asked to be on the board of the YMCA when I was still in my 20s. Our YMCA in Encinitas had a very strong mission of serving children and families. This philanthropic mission aligned well with our practice. We have always leaned into programs for kids at The Drake Center, including Kid's Day, to showcase the practice and let children get a behind-the-scenes tour of what it's like to be a veterinarian. In addition, we fundraise annually to help pay for training a guide dog for an autistic child. The impact these dogs have on the child and the entire family is amazing, and helping this group was a very mission-driven experience for my whole team.

Our doctors are intimately connected to diverse aspects of our community. Dr. Shotwell, for instance, is deeply involved in the equestrian community, with connections that extend beyond the confines of our clinic. Dr. Borsack grew up in Encinitas, and her character alone has attracted many family members and friends to the practice. They assume correctly that if she works at The Drake

Center, it must be a very ethical and great veterinary hospital. Each of our doctors is an extension of our practice in the community, and they reflect a lot about who we are and how we practice with integrity and compassion.

Challenges and Triumphs in the Digital Age

Digital communications took an unexpected turn with the rise of hyperlocal platforms like Nextdoor. While these spaces can be a valuable avenue for community discussion, they also pose challenges for business owners. One bizarre incident involved false claims against The Drake Center – an unwarranted attack that required careful management and a swift response. An employee from another hospital posted that one of our technicians was removed in handcuffs by the police. The funny thing was that we were open, and some people called to let us know about this false post. We did have one of our techs respond that this was, of course, false, and we asked Nextdoor to remove it. In addition, I called the hospital of the person who made the post and let the owner know that her employee had done this. I would let her handle the situation in her own hospital.

Navigating such digital spaces and responding to negativity and criticism[3] demands a delicate balance. As we address the need to be aware of online conversations, we also emphasize the importance of maintaining professional boundaries. Unsubstantiated claims, as we encountered, can quickly be broadcast to a large audience.

Our approach to managing these challenges involves maintaining vigilance without letting negativity seep into the core of our practice. We have an employee who helps to manage our marketing and media. She is responsible for monitoring the many online platforms and social media. Next, we have a team in the practice that includes our manager and two of our long-time employees who review each situation, decide how (or if) we should respond, including a doctor when necessary; we respond, and then we put it to bed. Once we handle a review or a platform, we move on.

The Outsourcing Dilemma

Many veterinarians, uncomfortable with the nuances of marketing, opt to outsource the task entirely. It's a common sentiment: "I don't want to deal with it; just do it for me." Unfortunately, this approach often leads to disappointment. Marketing companies, sensing the practice owner's discomfort with marketing, swoop in with promises of comprehensive services for a small monthly fee. It's a tempting proposition, but the reality is that, without active participation from the veterinarian and their team, these efforts yield minimal results.

This phenomenon is one reason I became a founding partner in a company committed to taking a different approach. We believe in empowering veterinarians to take an active role in their marketing. While you definitely need some parts of the work to be done by an outside team – you're not going to build your own website or create your own SEO strategy – you need to be an integral part of the process. After all, how can a marketing company effectively communicate who you are and what you do without your active involvement?

In today's digital age, people crave authenticity and connection,[4] even in veterinary practice. Your website and social media channels serve as virtual extensions of your practice, offering glimpses into your world when clients aren't physically present.

Does this mean that I am responsible for all of our marketing? Absolutely not. However, I am responsible for providing the time, resources, and personnel so this job can be done well. I meet monthly with my manager, our marketing assistant, and our digital marketing company. I am involved with their plans and activities, but I do not do them myself. I do, however, help provide content by way of videos for client information. In total, my contribution to our marketing is approximately two to three hours per month.

When clients aren't within the walls of your practice or on the other end of a phone call, your website and social media become the lifelines of communication. Neglecting these channels means missing out on opportunities to connect, educate, and build lasting relationships.

Building Trust Through Communication and Branding

The impact of veterinary marketing extends beyond promotion – it's a critical component of building trust, fostering connections, and influencing treatment acceptance.

Picture this: You visit a website, and it feels like a static relic of the past, untouched and disconnected from the vibrant energy of the hospital it represents. I've often found that an outdated website creates a noticeable disconnect – like pulling up a website in July and seeing the Christmas hours posted on the main page. In the digital age, our online presence is an extension of our practice, and, if our website isn't up to date, it can communicate to visitors that our *practice* isn't up to date, either. This realization prompted us to consider innovative ways to use our website, such as housing client handouts and videos. Imagine having access to valuable information at any time, even at 10 o'clock at night. This ensures that our clients feel supported beyond the clinic's physical walls and increases their trust in our practice.

Dealing with Dr. Google

As you've probably noticed, many people today seem to trust Google more than the medical professional in front of them. It's frustrating, but there is a solution. Here's a recent story that illustrates exactly how peoples' attitudes have changed – and what you can do about it as a practice.

One of our doctors was in the exam room with a client who had a possibly diabetic cat. The client asked the doctor, "What exactly is the blood sugar range for a normal cat?" The doctor responded that it's between 80 and 120 mg/dL. The client then proceeded (right in front of the doctor) to pull out their phone and do a Google voice search, asking Google the answer to the question. To the client's surprise, Google responded that "according to thedrakecenter.com, the blood sugar range of a normal cat is between 80 and 120 mg/dL." In other words, since our website is so highly ranked in Google, the answer her phone gave her was literally an answer from our own practice. Of course, it was very rude of the client to do this, but their attitude changed quickly when they heard the answer. Ultimately, the doctor and I laughed about this. We can be sure this client is unlikely to question our advice again!

Social media platforms are powerful tools here, as well. They're not just for sharing silly and fun moments – though those have their place. Social media serves as an avenue for education, providing insights into emerging health issues, and studies from multiple countries have identified behavior patterns where pet owners turn to online sources[5] and social media platforms like Facebook[6,7] to gain insights into their pet's health conditions as well as their preferred vet's opinions on trending health topics. Recently, we faced an outbreak of a mysterious upper respiratory condition, and our response wasn't limited to traditional news sources. We leveraged our digital channels to disseminate information, collaborating with organizations like CVMA to ensure that our clients received timely updates. We were also featured on local news to help quell the panic that other media were creating.

The Drake Center Experience

Our commitment to providing top-notch service goes hand in hand with the image we've cultivated. We've established ourselves as the Nordstrom's of veterinary care, a place where excellence is expected – and paid for. This branding not only sets expectations for our clients, but also plays a crucial role in ensuring we can charge appropriately for the services we provide.

An interesting incident highlighted the impact of our luxury branding. A discussion about our practice on a local platform drew nearly 250 comments, with clients affirming our excellence despite acknowledging the cost. While some people complained about our prices, others quickly responded to tell them that our exemplary care is worth the price. The consensus was clear: we're not just expensive; we offer exceptional value from the best doctors in a compassionate manner.

Crafting an Inviting Practice Environment

Over the years, I've had the opportunity to visit many practices. There is one common theme I have found in many practices without a clear mission and a brand: These practices are also often physically cluttered and unkept. My suggestion for these practices is always the same: decide who you are and what you want to accomplish. Make this a clear identity for yourself and your team, and then begin to craft your practice environment and everything you do to reflect this plan. It is amazing what decluttering a space can do for the clarity of what you are trying to accomplish within the walls.

When it comes to practice aesthetics, the saying "less is more" couldn't be more apt. A cluttered and chaotic environment can create a dissonance that permeates the entire client experience.[8] I've witnessed this pitfall far too often – cluttered counters, outdated décor, and an overall lack of cleanliness. In my view, a cluttered counter reflects a cluttered experience for the client, leaving them uncertain about what to expect during their visit. Addressing this issue is not just about aesthetics; it's about creating an atmosphere that aligns with our commitment to excellence.

Over the past 30 years, I've made it a point to continually update and refresh our facility. This includes everything from facility additions to flooring replacements and even reconfiguring walls to enhance the overall flow. The goal is to create an environment that not only meets but exceeds our clients' expectations. The practice environment is a dynamic aspect of our brand, and I believe that a well-maintained, inviting space contributes significantly to our clients' comfort and trust.

Our commitment to excellence extends beyond the physical space; it encompasses our staff and their appearance. Studies consistently show that clients have more trust and feel more comfortable with a healthcare professional who presents themselves professionally. In our hospital, we emphasize the importance of dressing well, reflecting the value we place on professionalism and the overall client experience. When our staff looks polished and our hospital exudes cleanliness, it contributes to the overall perception of value, reinforcing the idea that the investment in veterinary care is worthwhile.

Creating an environment that aligns with our luxury brand is not just about aesthetics; it's a strategic move. Clients are more likely to accept the value of our services when the entire experience, from the physical space to the staff's appearance, exudes professionalism and care. We are creating an atmosphere that justifies the investment our clients make in the well-being of their beloved pets.

While I understand the need for personal identity and expression, we're cautious about excessive jewelry, funky outfits, and so on. If this gets out of hand, we can lose the feeling of team cohesiveness, and this is felt by the clients.

Marketing, Recruitment, and Retention

Your ability to authentically market your hospital is very important in your recruiting efforts. Today, people moving to a new city explore potential workplaces through websites and social media.

So, your online presence plays a pivotal role. It's important to utilize these platforms to showcase who you are – not just as a veterinary practice, but as a team with a unique culture. By presenting an authentic image on social media and our website, you can attract individuals whose values align with yours.

When someone considers ten potential workplaces in San Diego, we want them to feel a specific connection with us. It's not about being the biggest or the loudest; it's about being the right fit for the right people.

Retaining a strong and cohesive team requires more than just competitive salaries and benefits; it demands alignment. Marketing, in essence, is an internal force, aligning the team behind a shared mission, core values, and the way we deliver our services. The key is communication, ensuring that every team member understands their role in fulfilling our collective vision.

Internal marketing has played a pivotal role in the success of my practice. It involves cultivating a culture where everyone, from the receptionist to the veterinarians, is an ambassador for the practice.[9] This alignment creates a seamless experience for our clients, reinforcing the positive image we project externally. The culture is reflected in our interactions, our services, and the overall atmosphere of the practice. This, in essence, is the heartbeat of our marketing strategy.

Marketing, recruitment, and retention are not isolated entities but interconnected aspects of a thriving veterinary practice. By focusing on alignment, we've created a practice where our external image matches the internal reality. Clients who experience this congruence are more likely to stay, refer others, and become advocates for our practice.

The Human Element in Marketing

One crucial lesson from this journey is the significance of having someone on the team who understands the consumer's perspective. For the past 15 years, we have had a role on our team that is the "marketing person." This individual is not a veterinarian or a vet technician; instead, they are someone who owns a dog or a cat and understands the client's perspective. This person bridges the gap between veterinary care and the client's expectations, ensuring that our digital presence resonates effectively. The role of our marketing person is to connect The Drake Center with our clients and potential clients via the myriad of online platforms.

Amidst the multitude of emerging platforms, from TikTok to Instagram, we have chosen a focused approach. We excel in areas where we have a strong presence, such as Instagram, Facebook, and Pinterest. The decision not to be on TikTok is intentional; it aligns with the principle of doing what we choose exceptionally well rather than spreading ourselves thin across every emerging trend.

Our website has seen updates approximately every five years, and we've incorporated video content to enhance engagement, as research reports that 54% of consumers want more video content from the brands that they follow and research[10] – veterinary practices included. The process of evolving and adapting is an ongoing commitment to staying relevant and meeting the evolving needs of our community. It's not about embracing every trend but about selecting strategic innovations that align with our mission and values.

Balancing Engagement and Business

In the era of social media dominance, finding the delicate balance between community engagement and business promotion is an art. Many perceive social media as platforms for posting cute pictures but, at The Drake Center, we see it as a powerful tool to keep our community connected while subtly reinforcing our brand and values.

For me, social media are conduits for maintaining a connection with our community. A significant percentage of our clients, perhaps 30–40%, actively engage with platforms like Instagram. By consistently sharing glimpses of our practice life, whether through adorable pet pictures or behind-the-scenes moments, we remind our audience of who we are and what we stand for.

Social media serves to present a strategic reminder, especially during those quiet moments at home. When a pet parent is relaxing and their cat or dog starts scratching their ear, they might find themselves on our website. It's during these moments that the connection we've fostered on social media transforms into tangible engagement.

While most of our social media content revolves around engaging visuals, we also recognize the importance of education. About one out of five posts is dedicated to sharing something educational. It could be a brief video, a link to an informative article on our website, or a snippet that imparts valuable knowledge. This strategic inclusion of educational content reinforces our commitment to not just entertaining our audience but also enriching their understanding of veterinary care.

Amplifying Your Practice Voice

The heartbeat of any successful veterinary practice is its team. Harnessing the collective energy of our dedicated staff at The Drake Center has been instrumental in amplifying our practice voice and extending our reach in the community.

While not every veterinarian may be inclined to create videos, I've found that tapping into their unique strengths is key. One doctor, during the quieter winter months, dedicates spare moments to updating our website and adding more handouts and information on new products or services. Another doctor enjoys creating videos and sharing insights and educational content. I often remind them that it's an extension of the conversations they have with clients in the exam room, a natural and authentic way to educate and connect.

Understanding that people consume information differently, we strive to cater to varied preferences. Personally, I prefer reading to watching videos, but recognizing the popularity of video content, we ensure a mix. Our aim is to provide valuable information in a format that suits diverse preferences, whether it's through videos, articles, or other engaging content.

Beyond the veterinarians, a subset of our team members enjoys the interactive world of social media. They have embraced the fun side of it, capturing candid moments and engaging with our community. Our marketing manager encourages them to be part of the content creation process, whether it's taking pictures with adorable pets or sharing behind-the-scenes glimpses. It's a lighthearted approach that not only showcases our practice but also allows our team to enjoy the process.

Creating a collaborative atmosphere is essential. Our marketing coordinator, for instance, doesn't just capture images but actively engages with clients, seeking permission to share their pets' stories. It's a symbiotic relationship where our team feels a sense of pride seeing their contributions shared on our platforms. This not only enhances team morale but also expands our practice's digital footprint through organic sharing.

Team involvement in marketing also creates a sense of shared pride in our practice. When team members actively participate in social media initiatives, it extends our reach organically. The ripple effect is real – when our team engages with our content, it amplifies the visibility of our practice within their own social circles.

The Impact of Marketing and Communication

Effective marketing and communication are tools that can reshape the dynamics for practice owners, pet owners, and the industry as a whole.

Overcoming Overwhelm

Practice owners often find themselves overwhelmed by the myriad aspects of marketing. The key is to recognize the fact that, like any journey, it begins with small steps. By gradually incorporating effective communication strategies, even amidst a busy schedule, practice owners can build a robust online presence.

Access to Cutting-Edge Information

The lesson here is understanding what aspects of marketing require personal attention and what can be delegated. While practice owners are the authorities on their clinic and clients, relying on a proficient marketing company ensures access to cutting-edge information and presentation, which is vital for staying ahead in the competitive landscape.

Presenting the Best Version

Marketing isn't just about visibility – it's about presenting the best version of your practice. By combining your unique insights with professional marketing support, you can showcase your clinic in a way that resonates with both existing and potential clients, fostering trust and loyalty.

Access to Diverse Educational Resources

Pet owners benefit from a wealth of educational resources. The diverse range of content, from case-of-the-month videos to national blog contributions, not only educates but also showcases the practice's commitment to disseminating valuable information. This access creates an informed community of pet owners who feel empowered in their pet care decisions.

Build Your VPOS: Action Steps for Marketing

1. **Define Your Mission and Values**

   If you haven't done this already, clarify your practice's mission, culture, and values. This will be vital in defining a great marketing program.

2. **Check Your Current Marketing**

   Now that you've updated and clarified your why (purpose), mission, and values, take a moment to look over your existing marketing. Ask questions like these:

   - *Does my website truly reflect the kind of practice I want to create, and does it show my mission, values, team, and qualifications?*
   - *Does my social media reflect my practice's values, culture, and brand identity?*
   - *Are my website and social media staying up-to-date with lots of new, high-quality content?*
   - *When I search for local veterinary practices in Google, does my practice show up highly?*
   - *How do my online reviews (number and star rating) compare with my local competitors?*
   - *Does everyone on my staff know exactly what our mission is and how we are differentiated?*
   - *Are we regularly participating in community events to spread the word?*
   - *Do my employees and clients regularly refer new clients to the practice?*
   - *Am I allocating enough resources (money and time) to my marketing?*

   Based on what you found in this evaluation, come up with at least three things you can do right now to move your marketing forward, and schedule time on your calendar to do this!

3. **Conduct Whole-Team Meetings**
   - Conduct a practice-wide meeting(s) to communicate the refined mission and values and make sure the team is aligned on them.
   - Connect this to marketing by asking team members how they can share this message with others and why that would be beneficial.

4. **Simplify Marketing by Knowing Who You Are**
   Simplify marketing decisions by solidifying your practice identity.
   - **Identity Clarity:**
     - Compile a document summarizing your practice's mission, values, and unique selling points.
     - Define the key aspects that differentiate your practice in the market.
   - **Audience Persona:**
     - Create a persona of your ideal client based on your practice identity.
     - Consider demographics, values, and communication preferences.
   - **Content Guidelines:**
     - Develop content guidelines for marketing materials that align with your practice identity.
     - Specify the tone, style, and key messages that resonate with your target audience.

5. **Partner with a Proficient Marketing Company**
   Recognize the value of professional expertise.
   - **Market Research:**
     - Research and compile a list of reputable veterinary marketing companies.

- Evaluate their expertise, client reviews, and previous work.
  - This should include specific, measurable data on the results they have produced for practices.
  - Ask for validated reports from third-party tools like Semrush and Ahrefs to show how they are driving traffic to their clients' websites.
  - Check the company's Google reviews and Glassdoor profile. Glassdoor is a website that tracks employees' feedback about the company they work for, and it's very valuable in this situation because if a company is over-promising and under-delivering to their clients, you'll see it in their employee satisfaction scores.
- **Consultation Meetings:**
  - Schedule consultations with shortlisted marketing companies.
  - Discuss your practice's mission, values, and vision for effective collaboration.
- **Decision Criteria:**
  - Develop a set of criteria to guide your decision in choosing a marketing partner.
  - Consider factors such as alignment with your values, transparency, and demonstrated success.

Marketing is not just an external tool – it solidifies the identity of your practice. The energy and time invested in marketing activities are also part of strengthening your overall business discipline. The effort you put into this area will pay off not only in more new clients (if that's what you're looking for), but in easier recruitment, stronger ties to your community, and a healthier workplace for your team, your clients, and their pets.

I hope that after reading this chapter, you have a better understanding of what marketing really is within a veterinary practice context and that you're better prepared to reach out to your community and show them what a great hospital you have!

References

1. Drake, M. Delivering on your mission while building a strong business. DVM 360 [Internet]. 2024;55(4):44–4. Available from: https://www.dvm360.com/view/delivering-on-your-mission-while-building-a-strong-business

2. Marketing Performance Study: Findings for Independent Veterinary Practices. GeniusVets.

3. Responding to Complaints and Criticisms. American Veterinary Medical Association [Internet]; AVMA. Available from: https://www.avma.org/resources-tools/practice-management/reputation/responding-complaints-and-criticisms

4. Medina, L. Authenticity as the Key to Success in Digital Communication and Marketing – MAU [Internet]. www.maufl.edu. Millennia Atlantic University; 2024. Available from: https://www.maufl.edu/en/news-and-events/macaws-blog/authenticity-as-the-key-to-success-in-digital-communication-and-marketing

5. Kogan, L., Hazel, S., and Oxley, J. A pilot study of Australian pet owners who engage in social media and their use, experience and views of online pet health information. Australian Veterinary Journal. 2019;97(11):433–439.

6. Kogan, L., Oxley, J.A., Hellyer, P., Schoenfeld, R., and Rishniw, M. UK pet owners' use of the internet for online pet health information. Veterinary Record 2018;182(21):601.

7. Kogan, L., Little, S., and Oxley, J. Dog and cat owners' use of online Facebook groups for pet health information. Health Information & Libraries Journal. 2021;38(3):203–223.

8. Moser, S. Minimal clutter, maximum efficiency in veterinary hospital design. DVM 360 [Internet]. 2019;50(6). Available from: https://www.dvm360.com/view/minimal-clutter-maximum-efficiency-veterinary-hospital-design

9. Drake, M. Internal marketing: how it can benefit your team and help you recruit [Internet]. DVM 360. 2022. Available from: https://www.dvm360.com/view/internal-marketing-how-it-can-benefit-your-team-and-help-you-recruit

10. An, M. Content Trends: Preferences Emerge Along Generational Fault Lines [Internet]. Hubspot; 2017. Available from: https://blog.hubspot.com/marketing/content-trends-preferences

10

Discipline

You're already disciplined in your work as a doctor.
Bring that same discipline to all areas of your business and you'll be set up for success.

Woody Allen has a famous quote: "80% of success is showing up." I take this to mean that if we show up to a scheduled meeting and we walk through a system of managing issues and opportunities, then we're already well on our way to accomplishing something good. When COVID hit, we had so many issues and opportunities to manage that I knew we would need a more disciplined approach. The Traction system was our answer. Our ability to move through our meetings efficiently was greatly enhanced by this system, and gradually we tailored Wickman's concept of an Entrepreneurial Operating System (EOS)[8] to become our own Veterinary Practice Operating System (VPOS). Having a disciplined

Veterinary Leadership: A Practical Guide for Practice Owners and Managers,
First Edition. Michele Drake.
© 2025 John Wiley & Sons, Inc. Published 2025 by John Wiley & Sons, Inc.

system for your meetings is a massive enhancement to accomplishing your goals. Showing up at the meetings is the only way to move your practice forward.

Meetings are, of course, just one area of discipline that's vital to your success, but as Woody Allen correctly pointed out, it all starts with "showing up."

The Discipline Behind Success

Growing up with parents who encouraged me to form my own sort of self-discipline allowed me to discover that I have some control over my life and certainly how I choose to respond. Discipline has been a guiding force for me that touches every aspect of my life and business. I find that often, it's what separates great practice owners from average ones.

In fact, I've found that most DVMs don't have much trouble being disciplined about their craft. For example, we follow the textbook formulas we were taught in school to prep a surgery and perform an OVH. But those same DVMs, when wearing their other hat as practice owners, will often fail to follow through in a disciplined way. This results in their business never reaching its full potential.

It's tempting to succumb to the daily grind and prioritize immediate tasks over the long-term vision. However, if you want to really reach your goals, commitment to planning and management is non-negotiable. It's okay if you need guidance on how to get started with this planning but it's not okay to not begin the process. Failure to engage in disciplined business planning will keep your practice and the individuals in the practice from reaching their potential.

Unless you skipped the rest of this book and started on this chapter, you've probably already realized that, in my experience, there are a lot of things you need to do outside the exam room or surgery suite in order to have a successful practice. This chapter is about how you make that happen, and discipline is the key.

In the midst of a hectic day of surgeries and examinations, of course, it's not possible to turn your focus to practice management, HR, recruitment, or marketing. It requires effort, time, and mental energy. Spend your days in the exam room and surgery focused on the patients and clients in front of you.

It's easy to be too busy and too caught up in day-to-day tasks, but it's precisely this mindset that hinders progress. Discipline helps us transcend the immediate emergencies (because those will always be there) and guides us toward a future where our practices thrive and our goals become a reality.

Running a Disciplined Practice

Always run your practice like you might have to sell it in six months. I've followed this advice without fail for over 30 years and the mindset that comes along with it empowered me to weather multiple financial downturns and periods of rapid growth.

You may be planning to sell next year, in 10 years, or never – but the discipline involved in running your business this way will make it a success no matter when you decide to exit. To begin, schedule the meetings. Block the time off for yourself and your key employees to work with all of the issues and opportunities that will allow you to get to the next level. This is a process and a disciplined approach to these meetings that will make a massive difference in what you can accomplish. And always remember "baby steps" because you will not be able to manage them all in one sitting. In the end, management is a process, and discipline will move the process forward.

This maxim applies to every single area of the business – but here are a few examples. It comes down to envisioning how a potential buyer would evaluate your business and taking the steps that would maximize its value in each of these areas.

■ **Pay Close Attention to Your Financials – Don't Let Them Drift.** Read your P&L statement and balance sheet carefully every month, and always know whether your profitability is increasing, decreasing, or staying the same. Meet up with your bookkeeper monthly and your CPA quarterly. You need these professionals to help you assess your business and plan accordingly.

■ **Know Your Numbers and Manage Them Carefully.** There are widely accepted benchmarks for a healthy practice that will allow you to get your margins to between 15% and 25%. If you find your numbers have drifted away from this, take a look at your operation and see how you can get back to the benchmark. This generally doesn't mean laying off staff or doing other extreme things – it could be as simple as delaying your next hire by a month in order for growth to catch up, refinancing a piece of equipment to reduce your monthly payments, or joining a GPO to lower your supply costs. **Having your key expenses close to industry benchmarks shows a financially disciplined practice, which will increase your valuation if you sell and provide stronger profitability in the meantime.**

■ **Have Disciplined Business Systems** so that a new owner could take over and the business would continue to run well. Don't make yourself the "hub" around which everything in the organization revolves because that greatly diminishes the value of your business and its efficiency. Any buyer knows that you'll eventually leave after selling, so if the business collapses without you, it's not really that valuable. **Having disciplined systems will increase your valuation if you sell – and give you a better lifestyle in the meantime.**

■ **Keep Your Business Growing!** Any business is either growing, shrinking, or stagnating. Nothing stays the same forever. If your business has made about the same revenue every year for many years, it is actually at risk because any external downturn could quickly push you into a nonviable range of income. This doesn't mean you need to grow at 20% a year – your growth should be appropriate to the demand and growth in your community and other relevant factors – but there should always be *some* growth. **Emphasizing consistent growth every year will enhance your valuation if you sell – and give you stability and confidence in the meantime.**

Building and running a disciplined practice doesn't happen overnight; it's a deliberate choice, often rooted in a combination of personal values, business goals, and an acute awareness of industry dynamics. Let me take you through the thought process and motivations that led to the establishment of a disciplined framework for our practice.

I feel strongly that people need to understand the "Why" behind what we do. This principle not only extends to our clients, but also permeates our internal dynamics. Having meetings for us is a cornerstone for discussing our objectives, dissecting challenges, and collectively arriving at strategies to move the practice forward. Like a shark, always move forward.

Creating a "Go-Getter" Mindset

Over the years, I've come to recognize that a focused mentality is very important to success in business. If you want to have more doctors, a larger facility, or new equipment, you have to put in the energy and drive to make this happen. It's a phenomenon I've observed not only in the veterinary realm, but also among the most accomplished business leaders. I would describe this mentality as including:

- *Ability to focus and have a clear vision*
- *High level of energy and drive in many areas of life*
- *Dedication and commitment to your goals*
- *Willingness to push through setbacks or challenges*
- *Discipline to stick to a plan even when it's tough*
- *Proactivity and self-determinism (the belief in one's own ability to take effective action)*
- *And never blaming setbacks or challenges on anyone or anything*

It's no surprise that many top business leaders also take on "bonkers" athletic pursuits, like ultra-marathons, triathlons, or mountain climbing. As a "retired" competitive downhill mountain biker myself, I recognize that many of the same personality traits that make a great athlete also make a great business leader. Focus and drive are imperative in any major pursuit.

What's the connection between these athletic feats and a disciplined mindset? It's a mental attitude that transcends both business and physical endurance.

But is this an innate quality or something that can be cultivated?

In my opinion, it's a little of both. Growing up, my father emphasized the importance of self-discipline, instilling in me an early understanding of its significance. While some may be naturally predisposed to a certain level of drive, I firmly believe in the elasticity of human potential. We can mold and shape our drive, pushing ourselves beyond our perceived limits.

My approach to setting goals has often revolved around self-competition. In all my years as a veterinary practice owner, I never worried about the competition. I am aware of it as a point of information. Instead, it is the drive and focus to continue to pursue our mission that propels our action steps. It's about being committed to achieving our full potential. I've always been curious about my personal limits and eager to push them – whether in work, exercise, or other aspects of life. I believe this has been an important factor in my success in business.

Pushing Your Own Boundaries

In my fitness journey, I often find myself pushing the boundaries, exploring what I, as a woman of my age, can achieve. It's not about being an "ultra-anythinger," but rather a quest to discover the full extent of my capabilities within reason. This mindset, intertwined with the discipline of maintaining a consistent fitness schedule, has had profound effects on both my physical and mental well-being.

As I navigate through different sports and adapt my fitness routine over the years, one thing remains constant – the energizing effect of accomplishment. The more I invest in my fitness, the more it fuels my overall vitality. It's a momentum that spills over into every aspect of life, reinforcing the belief that we can continually push boundaries and achieve more.

This infectious energy is a driving force behind my excitement for running my veterinary practice. Even as I embrace the notion of retirement, the passion for my work has never waned. The thrill of accomplishing new milestones, much like the thrill of reaching fitness goals, keeps the flame of enthusiasm burning bright.

Of course, none of this would happen without discipline. Like anyone, I have days when I'm excited to get on the bike and other days when I'm feeling tired or sore and just don't feel like it. But I've made a commitment to being consistent in my routine, and I know that I'll feel better after my workout – so I make it happen even when it isn't easy.

While I bring intensity and energy to my team, others on my team bring other talents that complement and enhance our capabilities as a team. We cannot all be energizer bunnies. We need the tried and true as well. I love working with all the varied personalities and traits of a team that leads us to our best.

Navigating the Challenges

Embarking on the journey of veterinary practice ownership requires more than just a passion for animals; it demands discipline and commitment. Unfortunately, not every practice owner embraces these essential qualities. In my years of experience, I've encountered veterinarians who, despite expressing a desire for success, struggle to implement discipline practices.

When I give talks about practice ownership, I often have practice owners come up to me after my talk and list all the myriad reasons why they "know they should do what I talked about, but they can't because A, B, C, D," etc.

To me, this boils down to a lack of knowledge and or a lack of discipline. If you're unhappy with your business and you know you can fix this by doing specific steps, but you're not doing them, how much sense does that make?

It's Simple, But Not Easy

Practice owner's often *do* know what they need to do, in a big-picture sense, but they lack the clarity on the exact next steps and the discipline to follow through and make them happen. Most challenges in a practice are conceptually simple:

- *I need to get my employees working together as a team instead of breaking into cliques between the front and the back.*
- *I need to have my DVMs give consistent recommendations so our clients will trust us more.*
- *I have a team member who is mean to the other employees, and I know I should fire her, but I can't find a replacement.*

You can think of a million more examples. The point is that these are all examples of things that are pretty straightforward, but they all require that you put time and effort into your business rather than staying "too busy" with patients to actually work on the business.

I recommend emphasizing action over excuses. Merely listing reasons for not pursuing a disciplined approach is counterproductive. Just as individuals with substance abuse problems must genuinely want to change before they can beat their dependency, veterinarians must be willing to embrace change and put in the necessary work before they can truly grow.

In reality, some individuals may not truly desire the transformation they claim to seek. The willingness to change and to endure the hard work involved is a prerequisite for progress. When I have people approach me after one of my talks and tell me all the reasons they can't do what I'm recommending, I can't help but wonder why they bothered to attend the talk!

Be Honest with Yourself

It's important to be honest and realize what you are (and aren't) willing to do in order to become successful. I have an amazing lifestyle today, but I didn't always. For many years, I worked six days a week and was on call the seventh day. I did this while also raising two boys. To say that there were difficult days is an understatement.

But, because I was so dedicated to achieving my mission and fulfilling my maximum potential, I maintained the discipline to push through on those tough days. And because I applied disciplined business practices along the way, it got easier over time. I built a strong team that supported me and helped us grow so we could all have more freedom in our schedules.

A genuine desire for change and a willingness to put in the effort are foundational elements required for your success.

Building Disciplined Systems

Over the years, our practice has evolved, and with growth came the necessity for more specific and disciplined approaches. I'll share a few of the systems that have been instrumental in propelling our success.

At the core of our disciplined approach lies a healthy organization and a well-defined leadership structure. The pyramid model, a visual representation of our leadership hierarchy, ensures clarity in roles and responsibilities. It's the first step in establishing a foundation that supports disciplined practices.

To maintain our disciplined trajectory, we've developed a systematic approach to our meetings.

First and foremost, we *always* have our meetings. The various meetings at The Drake Center are outlined in Chapter 4, "Planning." The discipline aspect is that we make these meetings happen, even when we're busy. We collectively recognize the importance of this, and we don't let other things get in the way. Remember, if you create a team, then even if you get bogged down, others on the team can carry you through a certain time and vice versa.

Before each meeting, team members compile a list of tasks from the previous session, outlining what was accomplished, what remains pending, and what can still be achieved. This pre-meeting accountability sets the tone for a dynamic and productive discussion.

During the meeting, we follow a structured format. Each team member quickly shares the status of their tasks – yes, it was completed, no, it was not completed, or any issues encountered. We refrain from engaging in detailed conversations at this stage, ensuring a swift review of individual progress. Anything that needs to be followed up can be handled in the issues discussion that follows.

Respect is another guiding principle that permeates every interaction within our practice. During our disciplined meetings, the atmosphere is characterized by a genuine respect for each team member. Whether discussing accomplishments, challenges, or issues, there's a shared understanding that every voice is valued, and disparaging comments have no place in our collaborative environment.

As we go through the yes-no statuses in our meetings, issues are flagged and listed on a dedicated board. Only after the initial progress check do we delve into discussions about the identified issues. This ensures a focused and efficient problem-solving session, preventing tangential discussions during the initial task assessment.

Completion is key, and every item on the list must be addressed. Even tasks lingering for several months are scrutinized, prompting accountability and resolution. This systematic approach ensures that all issues and opportunities are identified and effectively addressed.

The Ideal Decision-Making Model

To manage well, it's essential that you address issues openly and get full team support for the resolution. As Andy Grove[1] noted in his book *High Output Management*, the best process for group decision-making is:

1. Open discussion
2. Clear agreement
3. Full support

In other words, discuss the situation and all possible solutions; then make sure everyone is in agreement on the solution and the solution is expressed clearly, preferably in writing; and then everyone gets on board to push through the solution that was agreed upon.

Acknowledge the reality that not every issue can be resolved with a perfect solution. Sometimes, we need to embark on initiatives with a degree of uncertainty – trying new approaches or assigning tasks that require further exploration.

There's no room in a disciplined business for people to "sort of agree" in the meeting but then not do what was decided because they didn't really think it was a good idea. If team members have a disagreement, they need to be encouraged to voice it so that by the time we get to Step 3, we truly have the full support of the team.

By the way, it's not necessary for someone to 100% believe something will work in order to lend it their full support. Sometimes, you may need to ask your team to trust you on things, give it their best shot, and see if it works out the way you're hoping it will. Most of the time, it probably will work out, and your team's level of trust in you will rise. With that said, what you *can't* have is someone "going along to get along" but not really giving your idea their full support. This is a self-fulfilling prophecy – if the team doesn't take action to put your solution into effect, of course, it won't work.

Take Notes and Follow Up

During meetings, diligent note-taking is a fundamental practice. Document your discussions, decisions, and action items for various team meetings – doctors, staff, front staff, surgical team, and more. This disciplined documentation process fosters accountability and ensures that everyone is well-informed about the ongoing initiatives and strategies. Each person is responsible for taking notes on their own action items, plus what they may be responsible for sharing with others on the team.

Within 48 hours after each meeting, each team member should compile their individual lists and circulate them to the entire group. This swift follow-up ensures that everyone remains on the same page and can track the progress of each team member's commitments. It's a collective effort to stay organized, focused, and aligned with the overarching goals of the practice.

Cultivate Discipline Within Practice Culture

The disciplined practices we've instituted are a core part of our culture, and they represent our belief in working cohesively as a team. You can create a similar kind of teamwork in your practice through consistent discipline – when team members know they can rely on one another to follow through, they work together much better as a team.

Whether navigating challenges, setting quarterly rocks, or discussing individual tasks, a collaborative spirit should be in effect. This commitment to working together, coupled with discipline, creates a dynamic and thriving practice culture.

Discipline manifests not only in routine tasks but also in addressing challenges head-on. Whether it's a personal struggle of a team member or an unforeseen external circumstance, disciplined leadership demands attention and resolution. Once you really build this habit, you'll see that avoiding these challenges is actually undisciplined and unproductive. By proactively addressing issues, you can foster an environment where everyone feels supported and heard.

Communication and Flow Management

The heartbeat of your practice is the flow of your operations. Define clear roles and designate specific individuals to manage the ebb and flow of daily activities. In my practice, doctors and technicians collaborate constantly about schedules, patient needs, wait times for clients, staff efficiency, etc. We have an on-the-floor manager who is the go-to for the front staff when additional drop-off appointments might be added or an urgent case is on the way. In addition, this floor manager keeps the doctors on time by keeping their finger on the pulse of the business of the entire team. Whether adjusting schedules due to unforeseen circumstances or ensuring smooth transitions between appointments, disciplined communication will keep your internal dynamics agile.

Earlier, I recommended that you create an "accountability culture" – a culture in which everyone participates in maintaining accountability, ensuring that each team member understands their role in achieving your collective goals. From doctors to receptionists, everyone plays a vital part in upholding the standards you've set. Accountability is not wielded as a punitive measure but as a means of ensuring that everyone is aligned with our mission and objectives and works together in a disciplined way to achieve them.

As your practice grows, leadership shoulders the responsibility of understanding the progress of each team member, especially those in training. The leadership team actively seeks feedback, addresses challenges, and fosters an environment where team members can voice concerns without fear of retribution. This approach not only propels individual growth but contributes to the collective strength of your practice.

Aligning Systems with Mission

Every system we've implemented in my practice, such as the recent integration of online booking, was carefully aligned with our mission – unparalleled customer service. Recognizing that the world is evolving and our clients have evolving needs, we made calculated decisions to adopt technologies that enhanced their experience.

Running a disciplined practice is intrinsically tied to having a clear vision. As the leader, I've embraced a visionary approach, constantly refining my perception of what the ideal practice should look like. This forward-thinking mentality ensures that we don't merely react to industry changes but proactively shape our own way forward.

Selective Adoption of Technology

Discipline often means saying "no" to new ideas if they will not move us forward toward our mission – no matter how "new and exciting" the idea may be or how many salespeople are trying to push it on us. Sticking to your mission will always be your best course.

Online booking, for example, wasn't a trendy add-on; it was a calculated response to a tangible need, enhancing our service efficiency while respecting our clients' time. We often look at new technology and bat around ideas of how or why to use it only to shelf and reconsider later. Sometimes, it is just timing and how much a new technology resonates with our team. We also want to be aware of how many new ideas a team can effectively manage at one time.

Measuring Discipline in Your Practice

One measure of discipline in our practice is the ability to communicate effectively. This isn't just about conveying information; it's about setting the stage for understanding. Whether addressing your team or reaching out to clients, it's important to recognize the diversity of knowledge levels and perspectives.

For example, it can be tempting when a new employee doesn't quickly catch on to a task to simply handle it yourself and mentally decide, "I have to do everything around here!" This is a very common refrain with practice owners, and it gets in the way of growth.

The disciplined approach here is to realize that this new team member probably hasn't had enough training and to take the time and effort to get that training for them. Hopefully, you remember my "seven times" rule. It really does take discipline to keep going over these key concepts until people fully "get" them – but once they do, you have a stable person in your organization that you can build on.

In communication, it's also important to be disciplined about making sure that what you are communicating can be understood by the person you're speaking to. For example, not everyone possesses the same depth of experience or familiarity with industry jargon, so you need to make a deliberate effort to break down complex concepts. Before diving into the intricacies of a new system or procedure, take a step back and ensure that everyone is on the same page. And check back regularly during training to make sure everyone understands and is keeping up. It's *much* better to catch confusion or lack of understanding early rather than waiting for the person to mess up in a way that affects patient care or client service.

Discipline is also helpful in viewing discussions through different lenses – those of experienced staff, new hires, and clients. By adopting the perspective of someone unfamiliar with veterinary medicine, we can preemptively address potential gaps in understanding and better our training and information-sharing processes.[3]

Discipline, in this context, extends to our clients. We want to make every interaction, from scheduling appointments to discussing treatment plans, as straightforward as possible. This involves scrutinizing our systems, ensuring they align with our commitment to unparalleled customer service. It also means that we set clear boundaries with our clients and are disciplined about following them – this will come up in more detail in Chapter 11 on "Boundaries."

Avoiding Information Overload

Discipline means recognizing the threshold for information absorption. Overloading your team or clients with intricate details without laying a foundation for understanding can lead to disengagement. Strive to strike the right balance, providing enough information to empower without overwhelming. I have made enough mistakes in this area to realize that too much information is not a good thing. However, it does take some time and experience to find the right balance in sharing information.

Discipline in communication isn't a one-time effort but a continuous process. It's a recognition that, as the team evolves and new members join, there's a need to revisit foundational information. Regularly circling back to essential principles ensures that everyone remains aligned with the practice's goals and protocols.

Clarity as a Cornerstone

A disciplined approach also involves avoiding assumptions. What may be common knowledge for seasoned staff might be entirely new to someone just starting their veterinary journey. I recommend embracing the mindset that "There's always someone in the room hearing this information for the first time." This helps you avoid the pitfall of assuming shared knowledge.

The clarity and effectiveness of your communication sets the tone for understanding, engagement, and successful implementation of your practice strategies. If your team doesn't understand the plan, how can they be expected to follow it? And if you aren't disciplined about communicating that plan to them, how can they understand it? Keeping in mind our earlier chapter on accountability, if you, as the practice owner, can take responsibility for the discipline of ensuring your team fully understands and aligns with your vision and plans, you are on your way to running a successful practice.

Change Management and Accountability

Implementing changes within a practice is a dynamic process that requires keeping a keen eye on measurement and taking a strategic approach to addressing resistance.

Effective change management requires measurement. How can we gauge progress or identify areas for improvement without concrete metrics? In our practice, we embrace a meticulous approach to measuring changes, particularly those related to the introduction of new protocols or systems.

For changes that lend themselves to quantifiable metrics, we attempt to measure and review monthly. Whether it's the adoption of new diagnostic panels or the implementation of online booking, we count, track, and analyze the data. This disciplined measurement provides tangible insights into the impact of the changes, allowing us to make informed decisions.

I have been tracking my monthly new client information for over 30 years. Each new client is asked to let us know how they found us, and we have a spreadsheet showing where they come from each month. Knowing the total number of new clients and where they come from is a great way to keep on top of marketing and referral systems in place.

We use data each month in our leadership meetings to help us manage our practice. We usually stick to a high-level overview of KPIs, but we often evaluate other, more specific data when we are working on a specific compliance factor. For example, we may spend a few months educating or reeducating our teams about the importance of annual lab work and let them know our compliance goals. We then follow the lab data for a period of time to monitor our progress. If we are not meeting goals, we want to understand why and what else we might try to improve.

Addressing Resistance

Resistance often finds its roots in a lack of understanding. Our response is two-fold: education and accountability. When team members exhibit resistance, we recognize the opportunity to educate them on the "why" behind the "what." By communicating the rationale and benefits, we empower them with knowledge and help them independently decide to support the plan – not just because "their boss told them to" but because they really believe it's the right plan that will help us achieve our goals.

Discipline and accountability are inseparable. If resistance persists despite education, we shift our focus to accountability. Are team members following through on the changes they've been educated about?

Resistance to change is a prevalent issue throughout the healthcare industry, not just in veterinary care, and providing adequate support to gain understanding is crucial to mitigating resistance.[4]

For example, you might find some team members are resistant to recommending a particular medical protocol. When you talk with them, you might find that the root cause is that they are "projecting" their own financial constraints onto clients and thinking clients will not want to spend what it costs to deliver that level of care. When you encounter this kind of situation, make sure to resolve it by coming back to the practice's mission. Do your best to understand and acknowledge their concerns, respond with empathy, and then emphasize the "why" for this protocol – how it is the best standard of care and how that connects with the practice's mission. Then, help train those team members so they can be confident about communicating that value proposition to clients. In no time, your treatment acceptance will skyrocket, which will, in turn, help you deliver the best possible medicine and give you the resources to hire great team members and pay them well enough to retain them for the long term.

In navigating any type of resistance, it's important to strike a balance between upholding the conviction of the practice's standards and being flexible in accommodating individual circumstances. True discipline is not about being inflexible or taking a "my way or the highway" approach. It's about being so committed to the mission that, when obstacles show up, you find a way over them, around them, or through them – creatively figuring out how to best keep you going toward your goal. However, when we have a policy or a clear client recommendation, we expect everyone to follow this.

Navigating Finances and Upholding Values

Running a veterinary practice involves intricate financial considerations, often unseen by the team. Understanding the intricacies of a practice's finances can be challenging. Many employees really don't understand the finances of a practice, making it challenging for them to comprehend the rationale behind certain decisions. As a practice owner, I've recognized the need to bridge this knowledge gap.

To address this challenge, I periodically dedicate time to demystify the financial aspects of our practice. I've conducted sessions illustrating how a dollar traverses through the various expenditures. For instance, I help the team understand that there are specific benchmarks we need to adhere to, such as keeping payroll close to 40%. By keeping the payroll to a budget, we can plan for annual raises and hire more help as needed. A basic pie chart of expenses is also a good tool for employees to understand that when we charge $80 for an exam, most of that is used to cover our costs – it is not profit. Getting this information better understood can help foster a clearer understanding of the decision-making process and, hence, lead to more support for your decisions.

While financial transparency is valuable, I acknowledge that inundating the team with constant financial discussions can be counterproductive. Trust is fundamental. Our teams need to trust that we, as the practice owners, are committed to pricing services fairly. The focus remains on delivering the very best care, irrespective of financial considerations.

Be Proud – And Disciplined – About Your Pricing

The challenge of maintaining financial discipline starts with practice owners themselves. It's not uncommon for practice owners to grapple with self-consciousness about pricing, leading to a penchant for underpricing services or offering frequent discounts.

When you adopt the perspective that envisions selling the practice in six months, as I discussed above, this absolutely influences your pricing as well. Taking a forward-thinking approach necessitates a thorough examination of your practice's numbers, ensuring that the practice is valued appropriately. The key lies in striking a balance between fair pricing, value perception, and profitability. This may be a good time to lean on an organization such as VMG or to hire a strong veterinary CPA firm. They will be very helpful in making you comfortable with financial understanding, which leads to more comfort with charging prices that allow for a fair profit. A strong CPA will also help you keep your costs under control. If this is not our strong suit, it's good to lean on advisors who can help us to be our best.

Keep in mind also that, as I discussed in Chapter 9, "Communications," one of the most vital roles of your marketing plan is to support your pricing strategy by attracting the type of clients that have similar values to yours and are willing to spend what it costs to get the best possible care. When you're disciplined about pricing, if you find resistance to your prices (from employees or clients) and you know those prices are fair and based on the real costs of delivering great care, then, instead of simply backing down and lowering prices, you lean toward education and helping everyone understand why great care costs what it does. This protects your profitability, your brand, and the long-term value of your practice.

On a personal note, the commitment to profitability should also stem from the acknowledgment of the hard work invested in building and sustaining the practice. While every one of your employees probably cares a lot and works hard, none of them has taken the risks that you have in building your business; none of them cares as much as you do, nor have they worked as hard as you have. As a practice owner, you should be proud of this and insist on being rewarded financially for everything you've done to get to where you are today. A profitable practice isn't just a marker of financial discipline; it's a testament to the dedication and passion poured into the practice by the founder.

The Power of Education and Self-Improvement

Education becomes a cornerstone in the disciplined approach, offering practice owners and team members the tools to overcome challenges and navigate unfamiliar territory. The commitment to self-improvement is a key theme, with practice owners setting an example by actively seeking knowledge:

- **Seeking Information:** The disciplined practice owner actively seeks information through various channels, including books, articles, podcasts, and reputable business publications. This commitment to learning enables better decision-making and problem-solving.
- **Adopting Multiple Perspectives:** Recognizing the value of diverse perspectives, practice owners explore multiple sources of information. By considering various viewpoints, they develop a more comprehensive understanding of complex issues.
- **Application of Knowledge:** Armed with newfound knowledge, practice owners apply it to their unique situations. The ability to adapt and apply information ensures that the practice remains agile and responsive to evolving challenges.

Elevating Care and Service for Pets and Pet Owners

Running a disciplined practice elevates the quality of care and service provided. The systematic focus on refining internal systems and addressing management challenges ensures improved quality of care, better service, and happier employees.

Discipline in addressing issues such as team dynamics and unacceptable behavior contributes to a healthier workplace culture. Proactive management of cultural aspects, such as disallowing negativity, creates a more positive and relaxed work environment.

Discipline also means proactively seeking knowledge. Staff members in disciplined practices are encouraged to educate themselves continuously, fostering a culture of learning and growth.

Discipline emboldens individuals to confront uncomfortable truths within the practice so problems are addressed rather than ignored. By separating personal emotions from professional challenges, discipline transforms uncomfortable conversations into constructive dialogues. This allows for effective problem-solving without unnecessary emotional baggage.

By implementing the principles of discipline, practice owners and team members can experience a more balanced work-life, create elevated care and service, and foster a culture of continuous improvement and learning – all leading toward a more stable, valuable, and prosperous practice.

Build Your VPOS: Action Items for Discipline

Discipline is the bedrock of a successful veterinary practice, but understanding its importance is only the first step. Take concrete actions to instill discipline, and you'll witness the transformative benefits within your practice.

- **Discipline Self-Assessment**
  Conduct a candid self-assessment to identify strengths and weaknesses. Acknowledge areas where improvement is needed and be open to the process of personal growth. Ask yourself: Based on what I've read in this chapter, are you truly running a disciplined practice?
- If so:
  - How can you make sure this is maintained as the practice grows? What specific steps can I take to document what I'm doing and create accountability for my team? Write these down as an action plan.

- If not:
  - Name three areas where your discipline has been lacking and make a quick action plan to do something about each of them. Start with baby steps. For example, if you have not been paying enough attention to your P&L, start by committing to reading it within five days after the end of each month, and check your expenses against benchmarks. Doing this consistently for a few months will quickly get you more dialed into how to make the practice more profitable.

Discipline isn't a destination; it's a journey of continuous improvement and growth. Practice owners can initiate this transformation by combining self-awareness, team collaboration, effective meeting management, and a commitment to ongoing improvement. By taking deliberate steps today, you lay the foundation for a disciplined and flourishing veterinary practice tomorrow.

References

1. Grove, A. High Output Management. Vintage; 1985.
2. Drake, M. Veterinary Practice Culture and Staff Training: Aligning Your Team to Provide Great Client Service [Internet]. GeniusVets Marketing Education; 2022. Available from: https://www.geniusvets.com/veterinary-marketing/blog/veterinary-practice-culture-and-staff-training-aligning-your-team-provide
3. Industry Trends and Stats [Internet]. American Pet Products Association; 2023. Available from: https://www.americanpetproducts.org/research-insights/industry-trends-and-stats
4. Perregrini, M. Mitigating resistance to change in the workplace. Creative Nursing [Internet]. 2019;25(2):154–6. Available from: https://pubmed.ncbi.nlm.nih.gov/31085670/

11

Boundaries

Setting healthy boundaries is one of the most difficult things for practice owners to do – but it's vital to protect your well-being and your team.

As a practice owner living in a town where I knew no one, it was tempting to want to make sure my employees liked me, but I recognized that was not actually the most important thing. Of course, I wanted my team to trust and respect me, but I honestly believe that making friends with your employees is not a good plan. I genuinely like and care a lot about my team, but they are not my inner confidants. This is a boundary that I stress and recommend to all of my new young doctors. It's very important to have some people in your life who you can confide in for your mental health. Your employees do not need to know about your financial worries or your personal issues. Keeping this type of boundary

Veterinary Leadership: A Practical Guide for Practice Owners and Managers,
First Edition. Michele Drake.
© 2025 John Wiley & Sons, Inc. Published 2025 by John Wiley & Sons, Inc.

is so much healthier for them as well, because it prevents the workflow and environment from becoming clouded with stresses that these employees can't do anything about. If you are close to only one employee, it puts them in a strange and stressful situation compared to the rest of the employees.

Always be kind and respectful, celebrate wins and special occasions with your team, but do not burden them with being your confidant as well. Having healthy boundaries in our personal and professional lives can require some work, but it is well worth the rewards of good mental well-being and a healthy workplace.

When I look at all the different reasons practice owners have shared with me that explain why they are stressed or unhappy in their practice, I believe many of these really boil down to boundaries.

Practice owners and staff find themselves constantly battling frustration, whether it's between the team and the clients, the owner and the staff, or even between different staff teams.

The root of this discord often traces back to the absence of clear boundaries. It takes time as an adult and a business owner to understand boundaries in both our personal and professional lives. Some of us are lucky enough to have a great start of healthy boundaries within our families and how our parents behave. If you didn't have good role models growing up, then you need to take it upon yourself to learn more about boundaries and begin to create healthy ones.

As a new practice owner, there are so many decisions to be made. Having a clear mission and understanding the limits and moral stressors of both you and your team members helps to set healthy boundaries in the practice.[1]

A simple example of the importance of boundaries in my practice relates to employees bringing in their pets for care. We have a generous policy, amazing care for their pets, and discounts for our team members. However, we do require payment for services on the day they are provided, just as we do with our nonemployee clients.

By setting this boundary, we can continue this great benefit, be fair to all employees, and never have to be the "bad guy" following up to ask for money. There is a lot to running a practice on a daily basis. I do not want to add bill collecting from my employees to my list of things to do.

I've observed situations where staff members fail to comply with this policy, requiring me to step in and assert our boundaries. It's not about being the "bad guy" – it's about upholding the principles we've established for the smooth functioning of our business and ensuring they are applied fairly. If we let some employees run up a "tab" with the practice anytime they want to, it would become a whole project trying to collect those payments, creating frustration and stress for the team. It would also lead to unfairness, as employees who do follow the policy and pay their bills would most likely resent the other employees who don't.

When you create policies, it's crucial to enforce them consistently, whether dealing with clients or staff.

This does *not* mean you should be insensitive or position your policy as "my way or the highway" – you *must* take the time to ensure the staff understands why the policy exists. In this example, if an employee was wondering why we have this policy, I might tell them that our costs for supplies, doctor time, and equipment are exactly the same whether we're treating an employee's pet or a client's and that we are already greatly discounting these services for employees, so it's only fair that they pay their bill so we don't have to spend more time and energy collecting their payment. And, of course, it's not fair for some employees to pay promptly and others not to.

Remember, You Run the Practice – Your Employees Don't

Consider another example – the employee who consistently arrives late. Particularly with reference to millennial or Gen-Z staff,

I've found many practice owners simply can't figure out how to get these employees to show up for work on time.

This tardiness not only disrupts the workflow but also sets a precedent that can erode the team's commitment to punctuality. By addressing these issues proactively, we maintain order and prevent the build-up of resentment, fostering a positive atmosphere within the practice.

I've observed that punctuality and other related points of professionalism, such as adherence to dress codes, have really fallen off since COVID-19. I believe this may be a result of the tight job market, where many employees seem to think that they can get away with anything because they would be hard to replace. Whatever your dress code policies may be, you should be able to say so, and your employees should respect that.

It often seems like practice owners feel a bit powerless in these situations, either because they're not comfortable with confrontation or because they are afraid they won't be able to replace that employee who won't follow policy. However, in fact, boundaries are the bedrock of a well-functioning veterinary practice. If you allow your employees to walk all over you, you will have no end of stress as a business owner, and it will be much more difficult for you to achieve your business goals.

It's your responsibility to set expectations about these issues. Ensure that you clearly communicate these rules when hiring team members through your employee handbook, onboarding, and training. But once you've done so, you have every right to expect that if an employee has agreed to your dress code, code of conduct, etc., they should follow it. It's not fair for an employee to make you the "bad guy" by continually breaking the rules, so you have to keep correcting them all the time.

Whether it's adhering to payment policies, punctuality expectations, or any other established norms, maintaining these boundaries ensures a smooth and harmonious work environment for everyone involved. I strongly recommend that you have clear policies about workplace behavior and enforce them consistently. It's possible you could lose an employee or two, but those employees are not the ones that are actually making your practice successful, and setting this example will strengthen your culture and create loyalty with other employees.

Navigating Client Challenges

It's inevitable that you'll run into challenging clients or negative reviews. You can't prevent this, but you can decide how you will respond. When faced with such situations, our approach is to avoid allowing negativity to spread throughout the team and ensure the challenges are addressed, learned from, and then put behind us.

For example, I've observed a concerning trend in some veterinary Facebook groups and online platforms where a victim mentality[2] prevails. These spaces, intended for professional support, often devolve into complaint forums full of "horror stories" of bad reviews, mean clients, or bad staff. Immediately, dozens of others will chime in with their own bad experiences, and it generates a huge whirlwind of negativity. Like people slowing down to look at a car accident, you can be drawn into this content, which can undermine your enjoyment of the profession by emphasizing the negative.

In fact, these bad experiences are really pretty rare, so why do we give them so much energy and attention? If you had 99 great clients and one bad one, focus all your energy on the 99 and ignore (or manage) the one. There's no benefit to dwelling on negative situations anywhere in life. If a situation requires your attention, if there's something to learn from it, then handle it and learn from it. Beyond that, let it go, and don't waste time in online spaces that don't bring value.

I've chosen not to name these groups because I do empathize with why people might feel this way. But if you're in the industry, you've probably seen many of them.

I've also noticed a similar issue in these forums relating to work-life balance. While this is certainly important, I've seen a trend of practices almost celebrating the fact that they are closing earlier or not staying open on the weekends, which seems like the wrong attitude to me. Of course, individual team members shouldn't be working 7 days a week or 12 hours a day. But, practice owners can recruit and train a sufficient team so their practice can stay open when pet owners in their community need them, without any individual having to work an unreasonable schedule. If the practice is struggling to get enough people, the correct solution is to get serious about recruitment and training, as well as making the practice the best possible place to work so that people will want to be part of it. There's a lot of information in this book on how to accomplish this, such as in the chapter on "Culture," and there are many other great resources out there.

Handling Negative Reviews

Of course, it's upsetting to get a negative review. But when this happens, it's important to understand the issue, address it directly, and move forward with accountability.[3] There's no benefit to catastrophizing or indulging in a cycle of complaining. Remember, these reviews are not personal, so don't take them personally. If someone is ugly in a review, that means they are a sad human.

Here's a rough outline of how we handle a negative review at The Drake Center:

1. We address bad reviews as soon as possible.
2. Gather information about the case. Have a manager or lead team member call them to "hear their story" so they can get

this off their chest. Quite often, people just want to feel heard and want to know this will not happen again. Also, quite often, people have very unreal expectations. Either the expectations were not managed or the person is unreasonable. Usually, this call alone takes care of the bad review and many of our clients have later asked to come back to the practice.

   a. If we're able to resolve the situation with the client, if appropriate, we may ask them to amend their review to show that it has been resolved.

   b. Another option is to simply write a review response on the platform (Google, Facebook, etc.) that explains that we were able to talk with that client and resolve the situation.

3. If the person is unreasonable and rude, they are respectfully asked to find a new veterinarian.

   a. In this case, we would most likely add a brief response to the review platform expressing that we made an effort to resolve the situation and that the client chose not to accept the solution we had proposed.

4. Regardless of how we manage the bad review or a yelling client, once we are done, we pack this away under lessons learned, and we move on. We do not dwell on the occasional mean person or bad review. This again shows your team how you manage boundaries. Let's not let one tough incident dictate how the rest of the day will go with our awesome clients and patients.

Remember, when you're writing a response to a review, you're not writing it for that client – you're writing it for everyone else who will read the review later. If you are calm, kind, and thoughtful in your response, and the client continues to say crazy things back at you, this shows other people that the client is the problem, not your practice, and they won't worry so much about that one bad review.

I'm not saying every client is perfectly wonderful. After 30 years as a practice owner, obviously, I've dealt with my share of jerk clients.

But I can't change that client; I can only change the way I and my team respond to their behavior and try to create an environment where clients are encouraged to treat the staff with respect. This can be accomplished by building a strong culture. When your team is cohesive and supportive of one another, I've found that clients are much less likely to abuse the staff. And frankly, when you have a strong team like that, there are also fewer client service issues or medical mistakes that could open the door to abuse in the first place.

Boundaries in Medical Care and Service

One of the leading causes of professional exhaustion in the veterinary field is the lack of clear boundaries in managing exam rooms, surgery teams, and the front desk. When policies and procedures are not well-defined, some clients will push the limits. It's essential to handle such situations without anger yet assertively.

For example, the surgery team follows a carefully planned schedule determined at the beginning of each day. This involves considering factors such as the complexity of procedures, anesthesia protocols, and individual patient needs. It's about choosing what's best for patient care rather than succumbing to client demands.

Boundaries come into play when clients insist on specific scheduling preferences. For example, a client may demand their dog's surgery to be done first. In such instances, it's essential to convey that our decisions are guided by the well-being of the patients and not influenced by personal preferences. The surgery team's commitment to prioritizing patient care over client demands creates a sense of reassurance and stability.

By adhering to these boundaries, we uphold our mission and the professional integrity of our practice. The surgery schedule is not subject to external pressures but is meticulously planned to provide the best care for each patient. This approach ensures that the entire team remains focused on what matters most – optimal patient outcomes. When a client pushes back on this, and the doctor and staff respond with compassion but clarity, it reinforces our practice boundaries.

Fostering Support Through Firm Policies

Having firm policies in place not only streamlines the workflow but also provides crucial support for frontline staff, especially at the front desk. When policies are clear and unwavering, front desk staff can confidently communicate them to clients without fearing repercussions. This sense of assurance stems from knowing that these policies are established to ensure optimal patient care and are not arbitrary decisions.

When boundaries are firmly set, it creates a protective shield around the entire team. For example, when the surgery team is responsible for scheduling, front desk staff can relay this to clients without shouldering the blame if a client becomes upset. Knowing that policies are not subject to negotiation allows staff to express them courteously while feeling fully backed up by the established procedures.

Certain procedures and protocols, such as placing IV catheters or conducting pre-anesthetic blood work and pain management, are non-negotiable in our practice. These aspects of patient care are communicated clearly, and clients are made aware that adherence to these standards is mandatory. While these practices may require additional costs, they are fundamental to maintaining the highest standards of care. Clients do not get to decide not to have an IV catheter placed. This is a boundary in our practice, and it clearly communicates to our team how we adhere to our mission in everything we do. Obviously, things that are not yet covered by a policy will come up. In these cases, our team generally will make great decisions based on the knowledge of our mission, how we manage situations like this, and how to communicate with compassion.

Boundaries and a Positive Culture

Maintaining a positive work culture involves establishing boundaries that contribute to a productive and respectful environment. For example, fostering a fun atmosphere is encouraged, but we do discourage excessive chit-chat that disrupts workflow.

Another related boundary is our prohibition of gossiping about fellow team members. This includes refraining from sharing negative opinions or criticisms about a team member's performance. Instead, if a team member sees someone struggling or doing something the wrong way, they are encouraged to help the person out or, if necessary, refer the matter to a manager for further training rather than complain to co-workers about it.

The same thing applies to client interactions. Judging or criticizing clients is counterproductive and against our practice's values. It's essential to cultivate an environment where team members focus on providing the best care to clients without engaging in unnecessary judgment or gossip.

Managing Boundary Challenges

When boundaries are challenged, it's vital to address the issue directly. For instance, if a team member begins gossiping about another colleague's mistakes, the response is clear – bring it to the leadership's attention. The emphasis is on resolving issues constructively, whether through additional training or necessary interventions, rather than fostering a negative environment.

Upholding these boundaries requires accountability. Team members are encouraged to voice concerns through appropriate channels, such as expressing the need for additional training or addressing challenges with colleagues directly. By fostering an atmosphere of accountability, we ensure that everyone understands the professional standards that contribute to the overall success of our veterinary practice.

Managing boundary challenges is about fostering a workplace where team members feel empowered to address issues constructively. By emphasizing open communication, professionalism, and confidentiality, we create an atmosphere where boundaries are respected and everyone contributes to a positive and supportive veterinary practice.

Communicating the "Why"

To discourage gossip and negative talk, it's important to explain the reasons behind the established boundaries and enforced policies.[4] Team members may not have considered the impact of their actions on workplace dynamics. We have many young employees who have never worked in a healthy work environment. It's up to us to provide a healthy workplace and help them learn the importance of their participation in making it a great place to work. By highlighting the fact that such behavior creates dysfunction, wastes time, and doesn't contribute to personal or professional growth, individuals gain a clearer understanding of why we have these policies.

A strong organizational culture is instrumental in curbing negative behavior. Long-term team members play a vital role in upholding this culture by informing newcomers about expectations and boundaries. In instances where a new team member doesn't align with the established culture, decisive action, starting with coaching and sometimes even escalating to termination in extreme cases, may be necessary to protect the overall well-being of the team and workplace dynamics.

Every conversation about workplace behavior is an opportunity for professional growth. Team members are reminded that adhering to established norms not only contributes to a positive workplace culture but also enhances their professional development. It's a collective effort to create an environment where everyone can thrive and contribute positively to veterinary practice.

Navigating Baggage in the Workplace

In our hiring process, our Practice Manager employs the art of open–ended questions to uncover valuable insights into how individuals manage themselves. This approach helps us gauge their compatibility with our practice's culture. Hiring decisions are based on the alignment of values and culture, with an emphasis on selecting candidates who will contribute positively to the team.

Our hiring philosophy prioritizes culture over skill. We firmly believe that it is easier to train for skill than to reshape someone's ingrained behaviors. This principle guides us in building a team that not only possesses the necessary skills but also shares a common understanding of our practice's values and boundaries.

It's important to realize that new team members arrive with their own prior experiences and baggage from their earlier workplaces. People accustomed to dysfunctional work environments may initially find it challenging to trust that our practice truly operates differently. It takes time for them to acclimate to a culture built on respect, collaboration, and clear boundaries. However, as they witness our commitment to these values, trust gradually develops, and they either integrate into our culture – or realize it's not the right fit for them.

Our Practice Manager exercises caution when hiring locally, especially from other veterinary hospitals. The concern is that individuals who have worked at multiple hospitals may carry accumulated dysfunction from their experiences. To mitigate this, we primarily seek team members who are new to the area and have made a deliberate decision to join our practice or those new to the veterinary field who fit our culture and want to learn and grow.

When individuals join our team with baggage from prior experiences, we sometimes have to un-train certain behaviors and reshape their perspectives. We had a veterinary technician who joined our team after working in numerous dysfunctional environments previously. My manager remarked that she wasn't too sure about this hire. The employee had a lot of rough edges, but she thought it was worth giving it a try, as she had a lot of great skills and was a really good human underneath her tough exterior. Initially, she seemed to have a chip on her shoulder and didn't fully trust our culture right away. Being used to passive–aggressive behavior, she often had a hard time believing that when people were nice to her, they really meant it and were not doing other things behind her back. But she eventually saw that it was real – she relaxed, her productivity increased, and she became a great employee.

Establishing Trust in a New Environment

We implement a three-month evaluation period to assess the integration of new team members into our culture. If, within this timeframe, they haven't fully embraced our values and boundaries, it raises concerns about their long-term fit. While we always try to coach team members and retain them if we can, we also recognize that certain ingrained behaviors may be too deeply rooted to be fixable, and that person may not work out.

Ultimately, our approach to hiring and team integration centers on fostering a positive and productive work environment. By prioritizing culture fit, training for skill, and being discerning in our hiring practices, we build a team that not only excels in their professional capacities but also contributes to the overall harmony and success of our veterinary practice.

Setting Boundaries Around Aggressive Patients and Noncompliant Pet Owners

Lately, we've seen an increase in aggressive behavior among patients, a phenomenon possibly influenced by social media portrayals of treating animals like toddlers instead of dogs. In addition, a huge number of people acquired dogs during COVID-19 when training classes were tough to come by. To make this even more difficult, it seems that many owners are in denial about their pet's behavior and the danger it could pose to our staff or other people. While acknowledging this reality, we recognize the importance of addressing poorly trained pets with a focus on ensuring the safety of both the veterinary team and the animals themselves.

To manage cases involving aggressive patients, we have implemented stringent policies. These include requiring sedation for certain dogs before they even enter the practice. This approach not only protects our team from potential harm but also aims to prevent negative experiences for the animals, which could exacerbate their fear-based aggression.

When it comes to noncompliance in a medical setting, there is far more available research regarding human medical compliance than there is for veterinary cases, especially those involving medication. There are numerous factors leading to pet owner noncompliance, ranging from absent-mindedness to conscious objection,[5] but we, as members of the veterinary community, need to prioritize working with our clients toward compliance or suggesting they seek out care elsewhere. By setting boundaries with owners and insisting that all aftercare and medication directives are followed, we can create optimal health outcomes for the animals we care for and avoid unnecessary friction with owners.

Communicating our policies and boundaries to clients is essential. We make it clear that the safety and well-being of both the patients and our team are our top priorities. Sedation is presented as a compassionate and effective way to ensure a stress-free experience for the pet, even if it may incur additional costs and time.

Ultimately, balancing professionalism and upholding boundaries is an ongoing process. It requires a commitment to providing excellent client service while prioritizing the safety and well-being of both the veterinary team and their patients. The ability to adapt to evolving client dynamics and maintain a collegial atmosphere within the team is pivotal in successfully navigating the challenges of the veterinary profession.

Let Your Team Help You Set Boundaries

Feedback from our team is instrumental in addressing complex cases. For instance, we had a particularly difficult patient whose behavior posed significant safety issues. The clients were great long-term clients, but they failed to realize how bad their dog's behavior was for us. The team brought this case to our attention, prompting us to collectively devise a strategy. We involve the veterinarian to make informed decisions on how to manage the situation.

Navigating Work Ethic and Work-Life Balance

At The Drake Center, we've found a unique balance between maintaining a strong work ethic and accommodating the need for work-life balance. With 11 doctors on board, we've devised a system that ensures optimal patient care without compromising the personal lives of our team members.

Our practice is open until seven o'clock every night, and our team is on hand until eight o'clock. To achieve this, we've implemented a structured framework that allows flexibility. Recognizing the unique challenges faced by working moms, we've created a system that allows them to choose between working two, three, or four days a week. These 10-hour days, which include an hour at the end for case management, provide full-time coverage. We highly respect the demands of motherhood and acknowledge that professional women can find suitable childcare solutions for the days they work. For moms on maternity leave, we encourage a three to four-month break and support their gradual return to full-time schedules.

Clear Communication of Expectations for Team Members

We communicate our expectations clearly, emphasizing the necessity of full-time days for effective patient care. Our approach is collaborative, and while we acknowledge changing work ethics, we prioritize the needs of the business to provide the best possible care for our patients.

Similar to our approach with clients, we present our way of doing things and the reasons behind it. While we respect the evolving work culture, we emphasize that, especially in the medical field, certain business needs must be met to ensure the well-being of our patients. We've created a supportive work environment that allows for flexibility within the constraints of providing exceptional veterinary care. This means that our doctors work full 10-hour days and do not leave for child care, but they may choose to work two, three, or four days a week and may request days that fit their childcare needs.

Our focus is to find solutions that accommodate the needs of our team while prioritizing the mission and patient care. By fostering open communication and understanding, we've created a work environment that balances the demands of a veterinary practice with the individual needs of our dedicated team members.

The Benefits of Establishing Boundaries in Veterinary Practice

Setting and enforcing boundaries in a veterinary practice can yield numerous advantages for practice owners, staff, and clients alike.

Reduced Stress

Implementing and adhering to well-defined boundaries allows everyone to navigate their roles with less stress. By confronting situations where boundaries are breached, owners can maintain control and foster a healthier work environment.

Enhanced Job Security and Satisfaction

For the staff, a workplace with established boundaries provides staff members with a sense of security and predictability. Knowing what behavior is expected fosters a more comfortable and less stressful work environment, ultimately increasing job satisfaction.

Empowerment in Decision-Making

Clear boundaries empower staff to make informed decisions confidently. When they understand how the business handles various situations, they can navigate challenges with assurance, contributing to a more efficient and harmonious workplace.

Assurance of Best Care Practices

For your clients and their pets, thoughtful boundaries in your practice translate to a commitment to providing the best possible care. Clients coming to the practice can trust that your decisions, from surgeries to anesthesia protocols, are solely based on what is optimal for the well-being of the patient.

Consistency and Transparency

When clients are aware of the practice's commitment to maintaining boundaries, they can expect consistent, transparent practices. This transparency builds trust and contributes to positive reviews that highlight the practice's dedication to unparalleled care, even if misconceptions about pricing may arise.

Build Your VPOS: Action Steps on Boundaries

Assess Your Practice's Boundaries

After reading this chapter, consider whether you may have boundary issues in your practice. Here are some example questions you can ask yourself:

- Do you ever feel a bit powerless in managing employees or feel taken advantage of?
- As the practice owner, do you have a great lifestyle, or do you work longer hours than any other employee, often taking on work that should be done by others?
- Do you or your team members struggle with handling difficult clients?
- When you have an upset client or a negative review, do you manage it and move on, or does that negative energy stick around for a few days, throwing off the harmony of the practice?
- Do you have a consistent set of medical guidelines and administrative processes that you always follow, even when clients ask us to change them at their preference?

Based on your answers to these questions, consider implementing some or all of the following steps.

Team Behavior Boundaries

For any team members who have behavioral issues, make a brief action plan to address them.

- Commit to the idea that team members will either (a) adhere to the practice's code of conduct, including rules about dress code, punctuality, and professionalism – or (b) they will need to find employment elsewhere. There is no option (c) of continuing to work in the practice while ignoring the rules, as this breaks down the unity of the practice. Get comfortable with this idea and be willing to be firm – it will pay off enormously for you.

- Make sure that your specific policies are clearly spelled out in writing and that all employees are trained on them. This is essential because it's very difficult (and potentially unfair) to discipline an employee for failing to follow a policy that was not clearly articulated to them first. This includes, but is not limited to:
  - Dress code (including any rules on uniforms, visible tattoos, body piercings, hairstyles, and so on)
  - Scheduling and punctuality
  - Behavioral and cultural values
  - Communication norms and manners
- Once you've ensured that these policies are in place, carefully observe your practice for the next week or two:
  - Grab a notepad and note down instances where people are not following these policies.
  - You'll likely spot a few "serial offenders." Take these individuals aside (or work with their direct manager if it isn't you) and review the relevant policies with them. Set clear expectations of when you expect them to be fully compliant with the policy, and follow up regularly. Put your agreements with this person in writing if appropriate to ensure they take it seriously.
  - If that employee improves, validate and acknowledge them strongly (and publicly, if appropriate) so they really feel appreciated for making the change.
  - If that employee simply will not improve, terminate them. Of course, you'll need to follow all appropriate HR guidelines, such as written warnings. I'm not

an attorney, and this is not a book on HR law, but at the end of the day, you generally have the right to terminate an employee who consistently refuses to follow company policy.

- If you do have to terminate an employee in order to establish these boundaries, be honest with the rest of the group. Don't bad-mouth the employee, but do let people know that the employee was terminated because they were not willing to follow policy. This shows the team you're serious about creating a healthy workplace and will not tolerate behavior that undermines it – and this will actually improve the morale and engagement of the rest of your team.

Scheduling Boundaries

- **Shift Structure:** Create an official shift structure for your practice. Wherever possible, eliminate arbitrary random shifts, such as "Jane only works from 1:30 to 4:15 p.m. on Tuesdays."
  - What is the preferred shift structure for doctors and support staff?
  - Are there any specific considerations for accommodating unique scheduling needs?
- **Flexibility Guidelines:** Determine exactly when you will allow flexibility and when you will require team members to stick to the schedule. Write this down, make it known to the team, and enforce it fairly for all team members.
  - Under what circumstances should scheduling flexibility be allowed?
  - Can you create specific pre-set options rather than having every employee adjust at random? (See, e.g.,

my earlier discussion of letting doctors have two, three, or four shifts per week, with 10 hours per shift.)

- **Standardized Schedule:** Implement a standardized shift schedule. Set a goal for when you can have this in place, such as within the next two months.
  - Collaborate with your team and practice manager to finalize shift structures, communicate the new schedule, and address any initial concerns.

Case Management Boundaries

- Consider how exams and cases are currently managed within the practice.
- Are there common challenges or inconsistencies reported by the team?
- Any activities (such as surgery prep) that vary greatly from one doctor to another?
- What elements should be standardized in the case management process?
- Based on the above, establish a standardized case management system. Set a goal for when you can have this in place, such as in the next quarter.
  - Conduct team discussions on case management, create a standardized protocol, and initiate training sessions to get your team aligned on it.

When you create and consistently enforce thoughtful and realistic boundaries in your practice, you create a healthier workplace. It's an environment that is more predictable and safer, and one that allows team members to continually grow in their abilities. This also leads to better medical outcomes and better client service as well.

References

1. Holowaychuk, M. How to survive (and thrive) in veterinary practice. In: World Small Animal Veterinary Association Congress Proceedings, 2019.VIN;2019.
2. Kets de Vries, M.F.R. Are you a victim of the victim syndrome? SSRN Electronic Journal. 2012.
3. Responding to Complaints and Criticisms. American Veterinary Medical Association [Internet]; AVMA. Available from: https://www.avma.org/resources-tools/practice-management/reputation/responding-complaints-and-criticisms
4. McNamara, M. 3 steps to end veterinary gossip [Internet] DVM 360. 2011. Available from: https://www.dvm360.com/view/3-steps-end-veterinary-gossip
5. Maddison, J., Cannon, M., Davies, R., Farquhar, R., Faulkner, B., Furtado, T. et al. Owner compliance in veterinary practice: recommendations from a roundtable discussion. Companion Animal [Internet]. 2021;26(Suppl. 6):S1–12. https://doi.org/10.12968/coan.2021.0029

12

Wellness

It's difficult to effectively take care of your employees, your clients, and their pets if you're not also taking care of yourself.

Wellness as a practice owner can be a struggle. Living a balanced life requires a regular evaluation. This does not mean that we should expect that we can have a balanced life all the time. I had my first son within a year of acquiring my third and largest hospital. I was not a cute pregnant woman and definitely not a well-adapted new mom. Becoming a mom was a struggle for me. I used to wonder at the women who would be out and about and looking beautiful and relaxed two weeks after having a child. They amaze me. I felt way out of my element as a new mom, and after a couple of months, I returned to work and began life as a "working mom." My ability to fit in fitness, sleep, and other kinds of self-care was

Veterinary Leadership: A Practical Guide for Practice Owners and Managers,
First Edition. Michele Drake.
© 2025 John Wiley & Sons, Inc. Published 2025 by John Wiley & Sons, Inc.

greatly diminished during this time. However, I trusted that while having children would rearrange my balance for a while, eventually, it would come back. And it did.

If you decide to embark upon practice ownership, you'll be working long hours initially. However, this too will change, especially if you begin to put systems in place that allow you to have a life outside of your practice. Life is a journey. Remaining well-balanced and maintaining our wellness is a vital part of this journey. Always have goals, and always be kind to yourself.

The Wall and Beyond

I vividly remember a turning point in my career. It was right after I acquired my third veterinary practice. This one was special – it became the heart of what is now known as The Drake Center. But the journey wasn't a stroll in the park. The building was in a sorry state – dirty and neglected. Revitalizing it demanded not just a financial investment but a monumental effort in time and energy.

Merging my existing practice into this new space was like choreographing a complicated dance. It involved combining two distinct sets of clients, integrating new team members, and also making the hard decision to let go of those employees who didn't fit our vision. The stress was immense and, I confess, it began to show in my interactions with my team.

I'll never forget the day two of my team members confronted me. They were right – I had become uncharacteristically short-tempered. Their intervention was a wake-up call. Acknowledging this, I did something I hadn't done in a long time – I took a break. Just 24 hours off, a brief escape to a tranquil hotel in Laguna Beach. It was a simple act, but profoundly restorative.

One funny story from that trip – in an attempt to unwind, I decided to try a martini – they always looked so elegant and sophisticated. I didn't expect that it would nearly knock me out!

I spent most of that retreat asleep, which was probably what I needed most anyway.

That brief respite taught me a valuable lesson about balance. Yes, there are times when you must push through challenges with resilience and determination. But never at the cost of losing yourself or diminishing the respect and care for your team. We must remember that our own well-being is not just a personal necessity; it's a professional responsibility. After all, we are not inexhaustible resources. Taking time to rejuvenate is not just important – it's essential.

Nurturing Wellness in Veterinary Practice

My journey in veterinary medicine has been more than just a professional endeavor – it's been a deeply personal mission as well. I've always believed in striving to reach my human potential and helping others to do the same. This belief started with my children, guiding them to become their best selves. But it quickly extended to my veterinary practice, where I see each encounter as an opportunity to positively influence others.

Self-awareness plays a crucial role in this journey. It's about recognizing your strengths and acknowledging your weaknesses. Understanding when you fail and being comfortable with that failure is vital. We all make mistakes, and sometimes, we act in ways we're not proud of. But the key is to apologize, learn, and move forward.[1] This principle has been a driving force behind my practice and my approach to life.

When I bought my first veterinary hospital, it was this mission that propelled me. It's about being the best person I can be and fostering an environment where others are encouraged to do the same. What does this look like in a veterinary hospital? It means creating a healthy, thriving organization. We in veterinary medicine are incredibly fortunate to have the careers we do – caring for animals and nurturing the bonds they share with humans. It's a beautiful and fulfilling profession, from the technicians to the receptionists and everyone involved.

Every day, we have the privilege of interacting with puppies and kittens, and helping older pets, like gray-faced labradors and creaky sweet old cats, live better lives. We're in a position to offer empathy and support, not just to the animals we treat but to their human companions as well.

However, there's a tendency within our profession – as well as other professions in a healthcare setting[2] – to focus on the negative and to adopt a victim mentality around the stresses and challenges of the job. This mindset overlooks the beauty and privilege of our work. We need to shift our perspective and celebrate our unique, rewarding careers. We must actively work toward making our workplaces healthy and supportive environments, and realize our worth as veterinary professionals. If we're unsure how to do this, we should seek guidance and tools from those who have mastered it.

Flexibility and Growth

In this industry, the conversation often circles back to work-life balance and the pressures of the job. It's true; everyone in a veterinary hospital has their limits. However, it's crucial to understand that these boundaries are ours to set, not to be dictated by external forces or challenging circumstances.

During COVID and other tough periods, I realized the importance of adaptability and proactive problem-solving. People often ask why I keep expanding the practice. The answer is simple: growth allows us to do more good. By expanding, we can share our high-quality veterinary care with more clients and pets.

Moreover, growth fosters a vibrant community of veterinarians. At The Drake Center, we now have a team of 11–12 doctors, each with their own set of skills and talents. They also have unique preferences and needs. For instance, one doctor loves her yoga sessions on Saturdays, so we make sure that her work schedule accommodates that. It might sound trivial, but these small considerations make a significant difference in our team's job satisfaction and work-life balance.

Being open seven days a week also offers our team greater flexibility. This approach benefits our clients too, as it allows us to offer more services and extended hours. Growth isn't just about expanding our physical space or client base; it's about nurturing creativity and camaraderie within our team and providing our doctors with schedules that suit their personal lives.

On a typical day, we have five doctors working – two in our annex, two in The Drake Center, and one performing surgeries. Over the weekends, we have three doctors on Saturday and two on Sunday, with surgeries reserved for weekdays. Our call system, which rotates every 10 weeks, ensures that we're available to answer client queries until 9 p.m.

When it comes to scheduling, flexibility is key. Our doctors can choose to work part-time or full-time, with full-time being four 10-hour shifts per week. They can select their preferred days and shifts, and we do our best to accommodate these requests. Whether it's a doctor needing Wednesdays off for family commitments or someone preferring a specific shift, we strive to meet these needs.

Through all this, I've learned that growth and flexibility don't just benefit our clients and their beloved pets. They're also instrumental in creating a fulfilling, balanced work environment for our team. By valuing and accommodating the personal needs of our staff, we foster a more positive, productive, and harmonious workplace.

Navigating Flexibility and Boundaries

One of the most delicate balances to strike is between flexibility and structure. It's about creating an environment that supports both the well-being of the team and the operational needs of the business.

This isn't a haphazard arrangement; it's a carefully crafted structure, offering flexibility within a set of well-defined boundaries.

For instance, we employ a lot of young female doctors, so maternity planning is always part of our lives. When one of our doctors becomes pregnant, we discuss their plans post-pregnancy. This conversation helps us anticipate and prepare, whether modifying schedules or hiring additional staff if needed. I remember when I hired my first associate, Kathy (now my partner), she became pregnant within the first month. Her initial concern was that her pregnancy might jeopardize her position, but my response was supportive – we'd figure it out together. And that's been our approach ever since: a commitment to flexibility and support, navigating each situation as it arises.

Throughout the years, we've faced various challenges, but we've always managed to cover every shift. During COVID-19, for example, our team's resilience and adaptability were exceptional. We maintained our operations without significant disruptions. If someone was sick, others would step in; we communicated through a simple text message. This mutual support and willingness to cover shifts are fundamental to our practice's ethos.

This approach ensures business continuity as well as a supportive work culture. Our doctors know that if they cover a shift for a colleague, the favor will be returned when needed. It's this spirit of teamwork and mutual respect that keeps our practice thriving. We understand that if one doctor is overwhelmed, it affects everyone, so we've cultivated a culture where stepping in for each other is not just appreciated but expected.

Balancing flexibility with structure is key to a successful veterinary practice. It is possible to accommodate personal needs while maintaining a commitment to the team and our clients. This balance has been a cornerstone of our practice, allowing us to provide excellent care to our patients while supporting the well-being of our staff.

Building a Team, More Than Just a Practice

In our journey at The Drake Center, the essence of our success is deeply rooted in every team member believing in our mission. This belief is crucial, especially when unforeseen circumstances arise. For instance, when someone needs to step in unexpectedly, it's not seen as an obligation. We are caring for our community and ensuring that no one misses out on the care they need. This dedication might mean sacrificing a personal day or altering plans, but it's done willingly because the team understands the importance of their role.

Regarding our working hours, I've always maintained a firm stance on the 10-hour workday. I've faced some pressure to shorten these hours, but that simply isn't feasible for running a solid, reliable business. My approach with our doctors has been consistent: work can be two, three, or four days a week, but during those days, commitments must be met. We plan schedules well in advance, so arranging childcare or other responsibilities shouldn't be a last-minute concern. As a business owner, I do everything possible to accommodate and work with our team's schedules, and this system has proven effective for over 30 years.

Our shifts vary, ranging from 7:30 a.m. to 5:30 p.m., 9:00 a.m. to 7:00 p.m., or 10:00 a.m. to 8:00 p.m. Flexibility in scheduling is key, but maintaining those 10-hour days is essential for the consistency and reliability of our practice. Industry leaders, such as leaders at the AAHA, have advocated for flexibility in scheduling, highlighting benefits for both practice owners and team members, including increased job satisfaction, higher degrees of personal freedom, and more committed and productive employees.[3]

However, there's a deeper aspect to our practice's ethos, particularly concerning the high rate of burnout and suicide in the veterinary profession. I believe one of the core reasons for this distress is the lack of a supportive team environment. In our practice, we work tirelessly to ensure that everyone feels they're part of a cohesive, supportive team. This sense of belonging, of being part of something larger than oneself, is critical for mental health and overall well-being.

When someone faces a tough day, receives a bad review, or encounters complications in surgery, the whole team rallies around them. This support system extends beyond professional collaboration; it includes emotional and mental support as well. As the owner, while I still make the tough decisions, having a team that I work closely with gives me and everyone involved a sense of support and camaraderie.

We spend a significant amount of time at work, so it's vital that we not only work well together but also genuinely care for each other. This includes everyone, from the doctors to the support staff. Creating a sense of belonging and teamwork isn't just beneficial for our practice; it's essential for the well-being of each individual in our team.

Balancing Personal Wellness and Professional Responsibility

There's this idea of doctors leaving early, say around four o'clock, for the sake of personal wellness. While self-care is vital, it's essential to understand it in the context of our professional responsibilities.

At The Drake Center, our approach to wellness involves understanding and managing what each doctor can realistically handle. For instance, a working mom might decide that she can effectively manage working two or three days a week. This personal decision-making is what I consider true self-care – knowing your limits and working within them.

Our hospital operates from 7 a.m. to 7 p.m., a schedule designed with both patient care and practicality in mind. Surgical cases often need a full day for both the procedure and recovery monitoring.

Moreover, most urgent care needs arise in the late afternoon or early evening as people return home from work or school. Being available during these hours is crucial for our patients' care and aligns with our mission to provide the best possible service.

I regularly check in with my doctors, at least once or twice a year, to discuss their schedules. It's a proactive approach, ensuring that their work arrangements are still suitable for their current life circumstances. If a doctor is facing challenges, such as a spouse traveling frequently, we discuss and plan adjustments to their schedule. This way, we manage changes without stress and ensure continued effective team functioning.

However, it's important to balance personal needs with our commitment to the practice. If we choose to be working parents, then we're expected to be fully present and engaged during work hours, with childcare arranged for our children. This isn't just about individual preference; it's about maintaining a reliable and efficient service for our clients and their pets.

Wellness in veterinary practice requires that you make thoughtful decisions that align with both personal capabilities and professional obligations. By maintaining this balance, we not only take care of ourselves and our families, but also uphold our commitment to the animals and people who rely on us.

Embracing Challenges

One of the core beliefs I hold dear is the idea of being your best self and encouraging others to do the same. Wellness, in my view, isn't about the absence of discomfort. In fact, all significant growth stems from facing challenges and enduring tough times. There's profound truth in the saying, "What doesn't kill you makes you stronger." Without these experiences, we don't fully develop as humans. Vulnerability, openness, and the ability to acknowledge our faults and learn from them are crucial components of personal growth, whether the challenge is spiritual, physical, or emotional.

As a business owner, taking care of my wellness is a multifaceted endeavor. Mindfulness is a key aspect of this. Whether it's through prayer, meditation, or simply finding moments of quiet, it's essential for clear thinking and inner peace. It requires discipline, but the clarity and calm it brings are invaluable.

Physical exercise is another non-negotiable aspect of my routine. I make it a point to work out almost every day. This isn't just for physical health; it's crucial for my mental well-being, too. I've learned that I'm not my best self without regular physical activity. While everyone's needs vary, finding some form of physical exercise that suits you is vital.

Nutrition also plays a significant role in my wellness strategy. What we put into our bodies profoundly impacts our health and mood. I'm not overly strict, but I do believe in the importance of eating healthily. And then there's sleep – aiming for seven to eight hours a night is a goal, though admittedly, it's not always achievable. Good sleep is foundational to overall health.

Finally, the importance of relationships cannot be overstated. A recent book I read, *Outlive* by Peter Attia, emphasizes this beautifully. It highlights how vital strong, healthy relationships with family and friends are to our overall well-being. Nurturing these connections is as important as any other wellness practice.

Wellness, for me, is a holistic pursuit. It's about challenging yourself, staying mindful, being physically active, eating well, getting enough sleep, and cultivating strong relationships. This approach has helped me grow not only as a person but also as a professional, enabling me to lead my team effectively and compassionately.

Wellness as a Cornerstone of Professional Success

There's often a misconception that prioritizing personal wellness means compromising the care of clients and employees. However,

I firmly believe that taking care of oneself enhances our ability to provide superior experiences for both our team and clients.

Veterinarians, like many professionals, can get caught up in the never-ending demands of exams, surgeries, and client interactions. It's essential to establish boundaries for our schedules and for the entire team. When we look at successful business leaders, as high-lighted in books like Tim Ferriss's *Tools of Titans*,[4] it's evident that many have rigorous fitness, nutrition, and mindfulness routines. These routines are integral to their ability to think clearly, make decisions, and lead effectively. In comparison, my wellness practices might seem minimal, but they're grounded in the same principle: self-care is key to professional excellence.

On a practical level, integrating wellness into a busy life requires planning and discipline. When I was a new parent, juggling full-time veterinary practice and business ownership, every day was a carefully orchestrated dance of responsibilities. My husband and I coordinated schedules to fit in fitness routines, family time, and work commitments. Admittedly, during certain life stages, especially with young children, finding time for self-care is challenging. But it's a constant goal to strive for balance and wellness.

Now, in the latter part of my career, I have more control over my schedule. I plan my fitness activities a day in advance and am unwavering in my commitment to them. There will always be excuses to skip exercise, but maintaining a strict routine is crucial for me. Earlier in my career, I had to be more creative, fitting in workouts whenever I could, even if it meant sneaking in a quick visit to the gym or running while my mom watched the kids.

As for promoting wellness among my team, I encourage healthy eating and discourage constant indulgence in unhealthy treats. We have "ambassadors of fun" at the practice, but I've had to put my foot down regarding candy and sugary snacks. I believe in leading by example, living in a fitness-conscious region like Southern California. Many of my doctors are avid athletes, participating in Iron Man competitions and ultramarathons. They serve as excellent role models for the team, showcasing the importance of physical fitness.

Our practice culture also reflects wholesome behaviors. We don't emphasize alcohol in our activities, and smoking is a nonissue in our health-conscious California community. I believe these choices and behaviors collectively contribute to a healthier, more productive team.

The Vital Role of Wellness in the Veterinary Industry

In the veterinary industry, the concept of wellness extends beyond personal health; it encompasses the overall well-being of the practice and its team. The general lack of awareness around wellness not only impacts individual mental health but also affects the functionality and morale of veterinary practices. Emphasizing wellness can transform a veterinary hospital from a place of chaos and stress to a thriving, positive workplace. A healthy organization is not just a benefit for the staff; it enhances patient care and client service and makes veterinary medicine a more fulfilling and impactful career.

Build Your VPOS: Action Steps for Wellness

1. Educate Yourself

Start by reading books on wellness and leadership in healthcare. Identify key resources that can offer valuable insights into creating a healthy work culture.

- Create a reading list. What are the top five books on wellness and leadership in healthcare you want to read?
- Discuss with leadership the need for everyone to take care of themselves in order to be servant leaders.

2. Lead by Example

Practice what you preach. Show your team that you value wellness by taking care of yourself. This can be as simple as adhering to a regular fitness routine or practicing mindfulness.

- Personal wellness plan
- What personal wellness habits do you want to model for your team?
- Outline your personal wellness routine and commit to it.

3. Encourage Open Communication

Foster an environment where team members feel comfortable discussing their challenges and suggestions for improving the workplace.

- Communication channel audit
  - Are there effective channels for your team to communicate their challenges and suggestions?
- If not, establish a method for open communication, like regular one-on-one meetings or suggestion boxes. Very important – when you open a channel like this, you will often get more suggestions than you could ever implement (including some very bad ones!). This is okay; it's better to know what your team's concerns are so you can address them, but do not feel that you have to take action on every suggestion from your team. Any changes to the hospital should be aligned with your mission and worked out thoughtfully with Team One.

4. Regularly Evaluate and Adjust

Continuously assess the health and culture of your practice. Be open to feedback and willing to make adjustments as needed.

- Develop an evaluation schedule to check in on wellness on a regular basis – quarterly or twice a year is probably good for most people.

- How is your wellness as the owner?
- Are you following the wellness plan you created
- How is the wellness of the team?
- Any changes that should be considered to improve wellness across your organization?

There's a misconception surrounding burnout that working less or distancing oneself from the business can alleviate exhaustion. However, in my experience, the reality is quite the opposite. Engaging with your practice, pouring thought and care into every aspect of it, should be an energizing endeavor. When you take care of yourself consistently, you'll have the energy you need to invest in your business and make it thrive. And the more your business thrives, the more resources, time, and opportunity you will have to create the overall lifestyle you've always wanted.

References

1. Wallace, J.E. Meaningful work and well-being: a study of the positive side of veterinary work. Veterinary Record. 2019;185(18):571.
2. Arif, Z. Time for nurses to drop the victim mentality and realise our worth. Nursing Standard. 2015;30(13):30.
3. Reeder, J. Flexible Work Schedules: Alternative Workweeks Can Benefit Both Practice and Employees. Trends [Internet]. Available from: https://www.aaha.org/publications/trends-magazine/covid-19-resources/flexible-work-schedules/
4. Ferriss, T. and Schwarzenegger, A. Tools of Titans: The Tactics, Routines, and Habits of Billionaires, Icons, and World-Class Performers. Boston: Houghton Mifflin Harcourt; 2017.

13

Conclusion

OVER THREE DECADES OF practice, I have gathered a wealth of wisdom and experience, insights that have not only shaped my professional path but also illuminated the diverse challenges and triumphs my colleagues in veterinary medicine encounter daily. My motivation for writing this book comes from my personal commitment to share this accumulated knowledge and offer guidance and inspiration to others in our field.

In recent times, the narrative surrounding veterinary medicine has been overshadowed by discussions of burnout and adversity. While acknowledging these challenges is crucial, my vision for the future of our profession is rooted in optimism and empowerment. I firmly believe that the realm of private, independent veterinary practice is brimming with untapped potential – a veritable oyster waiting to be explored. The essence of my message is a call to shift

Veterinary Leadership: A Practical Guide for Practice Owners and Managers,
First Edition. Michele Drake.
© 2025 John Wiley & Sons, Inc. Published 2025 by John Wiley & Sons, Inc.

our collective mindset to recognize and embrace the extraordinary opportunities that lie within our industry.

The responsibility of cultivating a thriving, healthy veterinary practice rests upon each one of us. It's not imperative to have all the answers from the outset. What matters most is the willingness to embark on this transformative journey, coupled with the determination to be the driving force behind our individual practices, shaping them into remarkable centers of veterinary excellence. This book is my heartfelt attempt to guide, inspire, and empower my fellow veterinarians to envision and create a brighter, more fulfilling future for themselves and the animals we all are committed to serving.

Envisioning a Thriving Future for Veterinary Medicine

When I think about the legacy I wish to leave to the veterinary industry, it becomes increasingly clear that the cornerstone of my vision is the cultivation of healthy, vibrant veterinary practices. This book, alongside my speaking engagements, is an embodiment of that vision, aiming to instill a culture of wellness and positivity in veterinary workplaces.

The heart of this transformation is the local veterinary practice. Here, in these individual clinics and hospitals, is where change and improvement can start. Each veterinarian, along with their staff, plays a pivotal role in creating this movement, fostering environments where excellence in patient care and client service is not just an ideal but a living reality. The challenges our industry faces are significant, but the power to overcome them begins at this grassroots level.

Reflecting on my own journey, I recall the numerous times my practice faced daunting challenges – the economic downturns of 1992 and 2008 and, more recently, the unprecedented global crisis brought on by COVID-19. These were not just professional obstacles; they were deeply personal trials that tested our resilience.

What became abundantly clear during these times was the indispensable value of having a robust, supportive team. A healthy organization is one in which members can lean on each other, drawing strength when it's most needed. In such a setting, even when one individual might falter, the collective remains steadfast, propelling the practice forward.

My aspiration is to see this ethos of collective resilience and well-being permeate every facet of veterinary medicine. If each practice embarks on this journey toward creating a nourishing and supportive work environment, the cumulative effect will be transformative for our entire industry. This is the legacy I wish to build – a veterinary community where challenges are met with solidarity and strength and where the career we have chosen becomes not just a profession, but a profoundly rewarding journey.

The Power of Vision and Planning in Veterinary Practice

I want to leave you with a compelling vision – a glimpse into the transformative power of building a healthy, self-sustaining veterinary practice. Imagine, if you will, the liberating possibility of stepping away from your practice for an entire month, confident in the knowledge that everything will run smoothly in your absence. This is not a distant dream but a very achievable reality.

The cornerstone of such freedom lies in our responsibility to create a nurturing and supportive environment for our team. Once you establish a solid team aligned with the core values and vision of your practice, your physical presence becomes less critical. Of course, your guidance will always be vital, especially when challenges arise, but a well-prepared team can handle these situations with equal adeptness.

This approach has profoundly impacted my life. By creating a great organization, I've been able to extend my contributions beyond my practice, such as mentoring other practice owners and writing this book. The benefits have been tremendous, affording me flexibility in my schedule. This flexibility has allowed me to be there for my family and pursue other passions. It didn't happen overnight; it required careful planning and incremental steps. Starting with hiring my first colleague after five years of intense work, I gradually reduced my days at the clinic, balancing practice management with personal life. This journey, spanning a decade, has been one of growth, learning, and, ultimately, rewarding life balance.

Now, if you're a veterinary practice owner, perhaps skeptical or hesitant about embracing these changes, let me offer you this perspective: Ask yourself: "Do I yearn for a better life? Do I wish for a work environment that thrives and provides the best care and service?" If your answer is yes, as I believe it would be for most, then the path forward is clear. It's about setting goals, devising a plan to achieve them, and being adaptable. Remember, the best visions are those backed by actionable plans.

By committing to this journey, you're not just enhancing your life; you're elevating the experience for your team and the quality of care for your patients and helping us to make this profession better – together. That, in essence, is the heart of my message and the legacy I wish to impart.

Index

A

accountability, 25–46, 128, 197, 198, 214
  action steps for, 44–46
  "baby steps," 31
  benefits cohesiveness, 36
  benefits of embracing, 43–44
  commit time to working, 45
  continuous investment, 42
  core concept, 27
  cultivating across team, 37–40
  cutting-edge care, 44
  effective planning, 43
  elevated patient care, 43
  embracing, 29–31
  enhanced success, 43
  establish regular meetings, 45–46
  fear of tough decisions, overcoming, 29–31
  hiring and training processes, 32–33
  impact on client experience, 40–41
  is best lifestyle, 46
  leadership and change, 36–37
  nurturing culture of, 42
  practice leadership, 31
  practice management, 31
  pursuit of excellence, 44
  ripple effect of, 35
  shared responsibility, 43
  and staff retention, 33–35
  take responsibility, 44–45
  technology and, 41–42
  and training progress, 46
  transparent communication, 44

Veterinary Leadership: A Practical Guide for Practice Owners and Managers,
First Edition. Michele Drake.
© 2025 John Wiley & Sons, Inc. Published 2025 by John Wiley & Sons, Inc.